W9-BRV-122

Wavy, Curly, Kinky

Wavy, Curly, Kinky

THE AFRICAN
AMERICAN
CHILD'S HAIR
CARE GUIDE

Deborah R. Lilly

AN AMBER BOOK

WILEY

John Wiley & Sons, Inc.

Published by John Wiley & Sons, Inc., Hoboken, New Jersey
Published simultaneously in Canada

Design and composition by Navta Associates, Inc.

The cartoon characters Berna and Lula are based on the author's original art.

A production of Amber Books, an imprint of Amber Communications Group, Inc.; Tony Rose, Publisher, Editorial Director; Samuel P. Peabody, Associate Publisher; Yvonne Rose, Associate Publisher, Senior Editor.

For general information about our other products and services, please contact our Customer Care Department within the United States at (800) 762-2974, outside the United States at (317) 572-3993 or fax (317) 572-4002.

Wiley also publishes its books in a variety of electronic formats. Some content that appears in print may not be available in electronic books. For more information about Wiley products, visit our web site at www.wiley.com.

Library of Congress Cataloging-in-Publication Data:

Lilly, Deborah R., date.
    Wavy, curly, kinky : the African American child's hair care guide / Deborah R. Lilly.
        p.cm.
    Includes index.
    ISBN-13 978-0-471-69534-9 (pbk.)
    ISBN-10 0-471-69534-3 (pbk.)
1. Hair—Care and hygiene. 2. Hairdressing of African Americans. 3. African American children—Health and hygiene. I. Title.

RL91.L64 2005
646.7'24'08996073—dc22

                                                                          2005023406

Printed in the United States of America

10 9 8 7 6 5 4 3 2 1

Contents

Acknowledgments

Special thanks to Kitt Allan, vice president and publisher, General Interest Books, John Wiley & Sons, Inc.; Carole Hall, former editor in chief, African American Books, John Wiley & Sons, Inc.; Camille Acker, John Wiley & Sons, Inc.; Tony Rose, publisher, Amber Books, for seeing the possibility; Samuel P. Peabody, associate publisher, Amber Books; and Yvonne Rose, senior editor, Amber Books; Wayne "Zoom" Summerlin, photographer; Terrie Williams, the Terrie Williams Agency; and Kelly Starling Lyons, author of *Eddie's Ordeal*.

I wish to express my sincere appreciation to all of my clients who have been so loyal to me for so many years and thank them for entrusting me with the care of their children's hair, and their grand-children's hair, but please . . . not their great-grandchildren's hair.

I would like to thank my cousins Cheryl, Janet, Karen, and Sharon, who at a very, very, very early age allowed me to play with their hair.

I am grateful to my little stars Quan, Armani, Boonie, Ashley, Alexis, Caitlyn, Kiara, my goddaughter Brittney, Michelle, Tina, Nova Tynashia, Ivan, Javon, Jessica, Lauren, Melanie, Whitney, Milton, Myles, Sequana, Sholisa, Trolisa, Shanay, Tesia, Tyler, Justin, Jalissa, Zack, Frank, Jaylen, Johnathan, Tanaja, Aaron, Krystan, Isaiah, Jordan, Sa'diyah, Salaah, Tarashia, Richard, and Jasmin and their parents for taking the time to pose for the pictures and for allowing me to use their photos in this book.

I owe a debt of gratitude to the Cleveland Public Library; for many years it has been an invaluable resource for me.

I would also like to acknowledge the contributions of the following stylists and salons in the creation of this book: Ms. Dee and Jeanina at Bouncin' N Behavin', Susan McMorris at The Braided Fox International, Alisa Williams at Double Vision, Tonya and Jesse at McLeod's Beauty Salon, Debra Clark at Mystique Hair Salon,

Karmer Sams at Nouveau Creations, Tracy Stephens at 2nd Round Knock Outs, Danny Allen at Sharper Image, and Andreena Marshall Visions of Drama at Hiawatha's.

I am grateful to Tanya Jackson, Yolanda Dixon, Latisha Guise, and Toyia Reynolds, my fellow hairstylists, who have inside and outside beauty and talent. To all my family and friends, especially my mother, Louise, my mother-in-law, Bernadine, my brother Buggy, and my nephew Deon for their unconditional love and support. And last, but most important, to my husband, Mychal. Were it not for your love, support, encouragement, and photographic talents, this would not have been possible. Thank you.

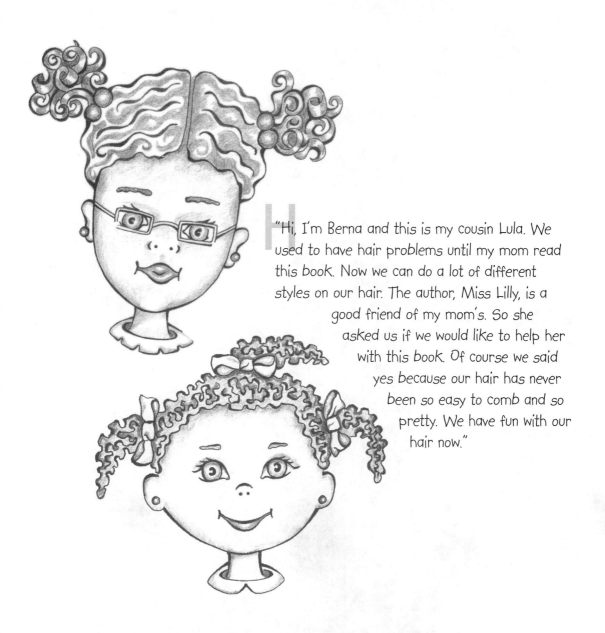

"Hi, I'm Berna and this is my cousin Lula. We used to have hair problems until my mom read this book. Now we can do a lot of different styles on our hair. The author, Miss Lilly, is a good friend of my mom's. So she asked us if we would like to help her with this book. Of course we said yes because our hair has never been so easy to comb and so pretty. We have fun with our hair now."

Introduction:
It's More Than Hair

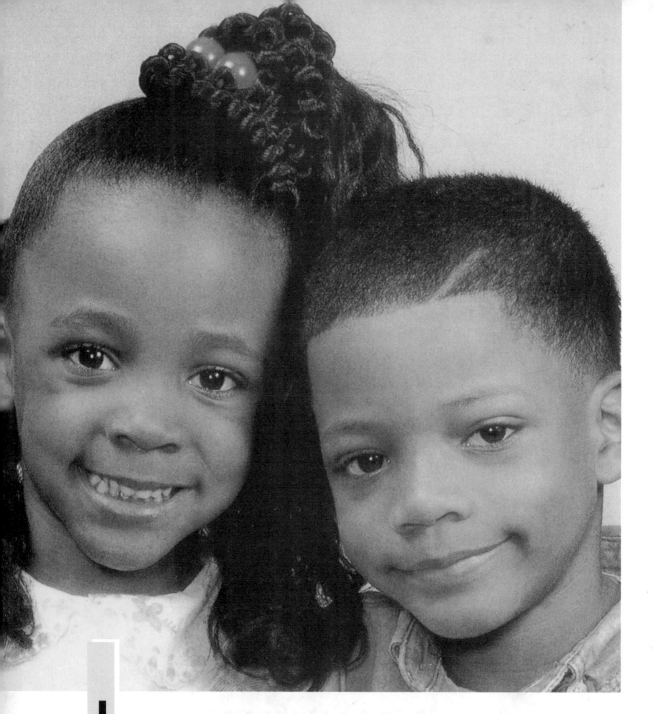

In some African cultures it was believed that the hair contained the soul. The hair, being the highest part of the body and therefore closest to God, was thought to be divine. The person touching the hair was important and trustworthy. Having created many strong bonds with children and adults through the act of hairdressing, I believe there's something somewhat spiritual that goes on during the simple act of combing hair.

Before we discuss the various methods of caring for hair, take a moment to relax, hold your child, and gently massage his or her scalp. Your special touch connects you to your child and reinforces the bond that forms between you and your little one from the very beginning of life. Children feel at peace and protected when you softly stroke their little heads while holding them or watching them sleep. They will feel cared for as you gently shampoo, comb, or brush their hair. Your tender touch can express love to your newborn and help create an inner strength in your growing toddler.

Some days doing your child's hair feels like a chore, especially on busy mornings when everyone is rushing to work and to school. On a Saturday afternoon, slow down and remember that time can be precious. Grooming your child's hair at any age gives you an opportunity to share some special moments. It's a great time to tell stories, hear about your child's day, or help her resolve any challenges she might be facing. You are showing your child that she means the world to you by taking the time to make her feel and look good. Your child will know that good grooming habits are important and that you are doing her hair because you care about her.

Wavy, Curly, Kinky: The African American Child's Hair Care Guide has been designed and written to help you take better care of your child's hair and to make the daily hair care routine a great experience for you and your child.

In my years of being a hairdresser I have tested and tried hundreds of different hair products and styles on children of all ages. There are no hard-and-fast rules, but I can share many proven methods. Far too often, I have seen African American children's hair in bad condition and known that with a little time, nurturing, and guidance the problem could have been avoided. Whether you need a lot of instruction or just a few easy tips, there'll be something in this book to help you learn how to take care of your African American child's hair.

I recommend that you use this book according to your personal needs. First, read the entire book and then decide what sections best relate to your child's hair care needs. Many times it helps to see a photo or an illustration. I have included pictures and technical photos so that you can see and better understand how to follow the steps that are discussed in this book.

If you feel the task is too overwhelming, seek the help of a professional hairstylist. Regardless of your child's hair texture and how he or she frets when you comb his or her hair, there are ways to make hair care easier.

We'll discuss hair care for infants and children up to twelve years old. The beginning of the book will focus on our young girls because, let's face it, they require more time and attention than our boys. At the end of the book, I have listed tools and products that will help make your job easier, along with a question-and-answer section called "What If?" I've also included specific instructions about relaxers for girls.

Read carefully according to your son's or daughter's age group and hair texture.* Remember, what you do today will bring about good or bad results tomorrow. Starting good hair grooming habits at the beginning of your child's life will make for a healthier attitude and healthier hair in the future. The rewards are great hair, happy kids, and delighted adults.

---

*In today's society, "family" is often extended to include grandparents, aunts, uncles, godparents, and friends, and you may be providing hair care to your child, grandchild, niece, nephew, or even a friend's child. But for simplicity's sake, I will refer to all children in this book as "son," "daughter," or "your child."

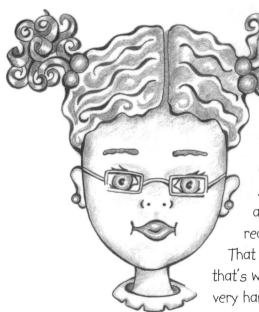

Berna:

"My mom said everybody has different kinds of hair. Some people have straight hair, some people have curly hair, and some people have hair that is really, really curly. My dad said his hair is nappy. That means his hair is super-duper curly and that's why he keeps it cut real short. He looks very handsome to me."

Lula:

"My mom said that's just the way it is. We don't get to pick what kind of hair we have. The best thing to do is to take care of it, no matter what kind it is."

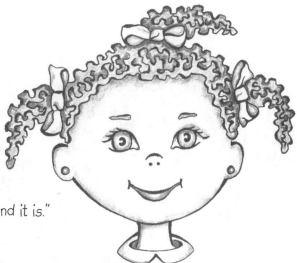

What Is Your Child's Hair Texture? 1

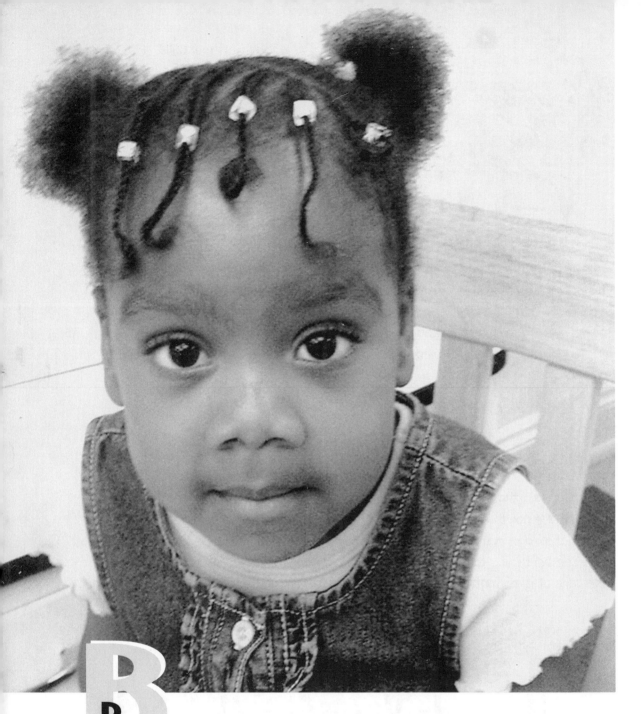

Before you try styling your child's hair, I want you to have a clear understanding of hair textures. Once you have figured out the texture of your child's hair, you can begin to use the right products, tools, and hair care techniques. You can then establish a routine for what I call "training the hair." It may take six

6

months to a year, but you will see a vast improvement in your child's hair, and maybe even in your child's attitude.

African American hair comes in different textures, which can be very confusing. But once you know how to care for your child's texture of hair, it becomes easy to work with. The textures can be classified into three categories: (1) kinky or excessively curly, (2) curly, and (3) wavy.

Your child's hair may be a combination of these textures or an extreme of one type, but the care of the hair will be based on these three categories. These textures also come in different thicknesses and lengths, which plays a major role in how you take care of your child's hair. Parents cannot predict the texture of their child's hair; it

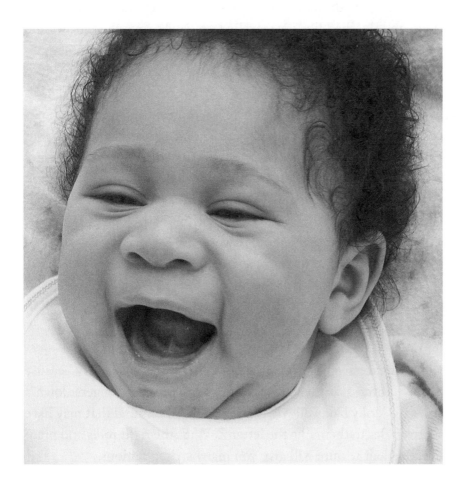

LESS STRESS

When you're styling your child's hair, the right comb or brush can mean the difference between laughter and tears.

has its own special genetic design. Sometimes you will also notice that your child has a different hair color from your own, but even that often changes as your child grows. The most important factor is that you recognize if your child's hair texture is changing and take care of it accordingly.

Your child's natural hair texture changes extensively between infancy and the age of four. During this time your child's silky smooth hair may have turned into a curly afro. Or, as in many cases, your child may have come into this world with a little peach fuzz and for about eighteen months had very little or no hair. Then before you knew what happened, your child had so much hair it shocked you.

Hair goes through three stages—the sleep stage, the growth stage, and the shedding, or recycling, stage. As your child grows and you comb his or her hair, you will see hair in the comb—sometimes more and sometimes less. On some days you may see fifty to a hundred strands of hair. If you see excessive shedding, broken-off hair, or patches, it could mean there is a problem, and your child may need to see a dermatologist. Pay attention to the changes in your child's hair.

Many of your hair care techniques will depend not on the sex of your child but on your child's hair growth, on the texture of your child's hair, and on how the texture of the hair changes with age. What worked one year may not work the following year, and you may need to move to the next texture or age group. Let's look more closely at the different hair textures.

Kinky Hair

Kinky or excessively curly hair has a tight curl. It can be dry because of the tightness of the curl pattern. If you run your fingers down a strand of kinky hair, you will feel bumps on the strand that may have sharp angles to them like the letter Z. With the right tools and practice, this hair texture will give you many styling options.

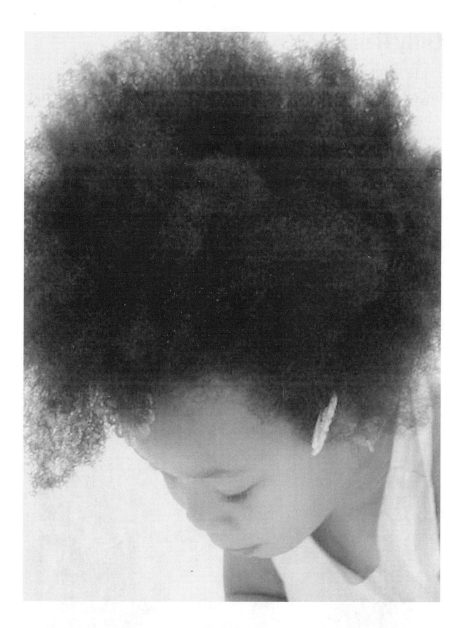

Unfortunately, people think kinky or excessively curly hair is "bad hair." It's not. No natural hair texture is bad, only hair that is not taken care of properly. Our kinky hair was designed by the Creator to absorb the heat and to protect us from the elements, which was essential for many of our ancestors, who lived in hot climates and spent long periods of time outside in the sun.

Curly Hair

Curly hair has less spring to it than kinky hair. When you run your fingers down a strand of curly hair, you will feel curves on the strand. The curls in curly hair come in all forms—ringlets, circles, loops, or even spirals—and the hair itself may be thick or thin, fine, medium, or coarse. As your child grows, the curls may change from tight to loose or vice versa. Curly hair can be dry or oily, so how you take care of this texture of hair is very important. Curly hair can become difficult to handle if the wrong products or tools are used, or if you overhandle it by brushing or touching it too much.

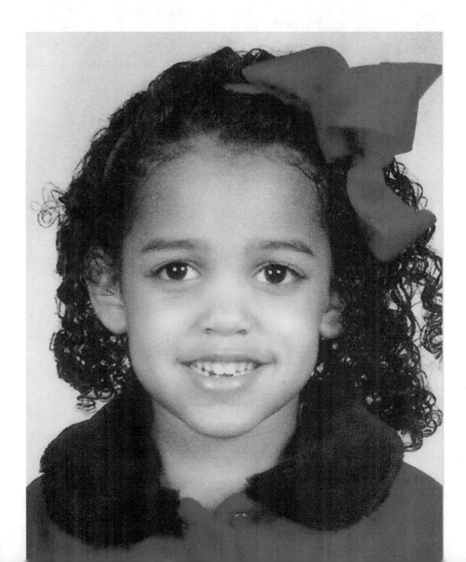

Wavy Hair

If you take a strand of wavy hair and run your finger down it, the hair feels smooth. Wavy hair has a silky look and feel to it. When you pull on a strand it springs back into an "S" pattern. This type of hair is usually very soft, especially on infants; sometimes children of multicultural heritage have this hair texture. Caring for wavy hair in the early years is not that difficult, but as your child gets older his or her hair may become curlier or straighter; it all depends on your child's heritage and how the hair is cared for.

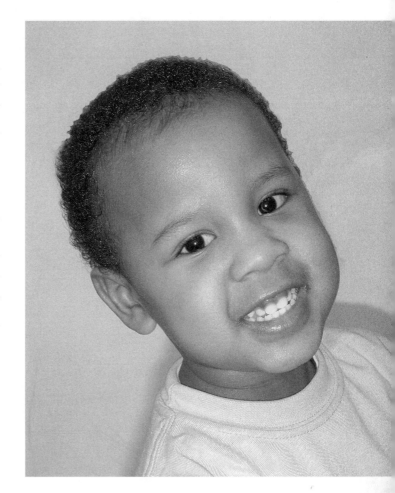

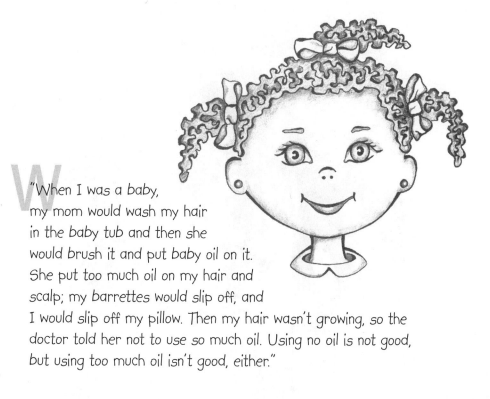

"When I was a baby, my mom would wash my hair in the baby tub and then she would brush it and put baby oil on it. She put too much oil on my hair and scalp; my barrettes would slip off, and I would slip off my pillow. Then my hair wasn't growing, so the doctor told her not to use so much oil. Using no oil is not good, but using too much oil isn't good, either."

Gentle Touches— Infants to Children Two Years Old

2

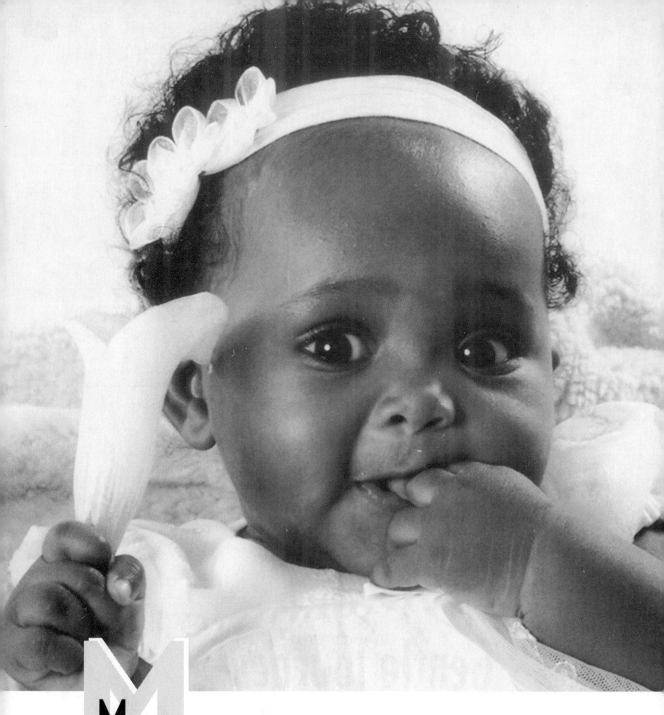

Many African American infants are born with very little or no hair; I call it "angel hair." It's so pure and new, but when that DNA kicks in, the true texture starts to push out the angel hair and the real hair comes in.

With infants, the styling options for boys and girls are often the same. What is more important at this stage is shampooing your child's hair every three to five days. To make it easier, the best time to shampoo your baby's hair is during bath time; usually one soaping is enough. For children who are crawling, two soapings may be needed. Make sure you test the water temperature first; you want the water to be warm. You should have your infant in a proper bath pad or seat. A child-safe water toy can make bath time more fun.

Use a mild baby shampoo designed for African American children, which can be more moisturizing than standard baby shampoo. To begin shampooing, dampen the hair with a white facecloth. Pour a small amount of shampoo into your hands and rub them together slightly; then apply the shampoo to your child's hair.

Using the tips of your fingers on the scalp, make small circular motions, then move your hands onto the hair and gently massage the hair. Make sure you never use your nails. Shampoo the hair in one direction; this causes fewer tangles. You should get a good head of lather; if you don't, rinse the hair and repeat the shampooing. Try to keep your child's head straight up or slightly back, depending on what he or she finds more comfortable.

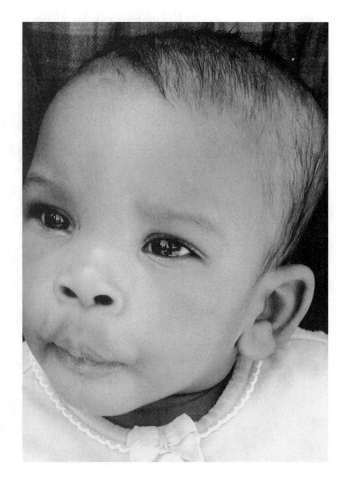

When rinsing the hair, always use a white facecloth and run clear water from the faucet. Rinse until you have removed all the shampoo from your child's hair and scalp. Next, towel-dry the hair in the same direction you shampooed. Use white towels when drying because colored towels may bleed dye onto the skin and the hair.

Infant hair care is fairly simple: you want to keep it clean and combed, and apply oil to the hair only if needed. You should use a light oil made for babies on the hair and scalp; as your child gets older you can switch to a regular light oil made for children. Brush your child's hair in the direction that it grows. This stimulates hair growth. If the hair is thick, comb it gently first, then brush it. When you do this, the hair will lie down better and may stay in place longer.

If your little girl's hair is long enough, it should be braided or secured with a safe hair ornament. Boys' hair can be left natural.

If Your Child Has Kinky Hair

Kinky hair can be difficult to comb when it is very wet because this texture of hair shrinks. Leaving a little moisture in it will help with

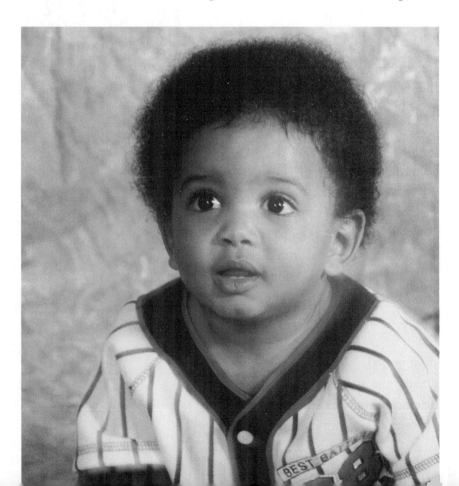

the combing process, but too much will only make matters worse. Apply oil to this texture of hair, massaging it into the scalp, not just into the hair. Massaging stimulates growth, but don't overdo it; too much hair oil is just as bad as not enough because it will weigh the hair down and make it harder to comb. Using too much oil also attracts dirt to the hair and clogs up the pores on the scalp, causing slower hair growth.

If Your Child Has Curly Hair

Depending on the length and thickness of your child's hair, curly hair has a tendency to tangle more than other textures of hair. The proper comb-out technique starts with the shampoo. Always try to shampoo your child's hair with your fingertips, keeping your fingers underneath the hair as you shampoo. Pat the hair gently to remove excess water and apply a detangling rinse as needed. Then, with a wide-tooth comb, take a handful of hair in the nape area and begin to comb it from the ends toward the scalp. Continue this procedure throughout the entire head. Once all the tangles have been removed, comb the hair from the scalp to the ends and apply a light hairdressing cream or oil to the hair and scalp. You can use your fingers or a pencil to coil the hair and create pretty, neat curls. Then let the hair dry.

LESS STRESS

Let curly hair air-dry whenever possible instead of towel-drying.

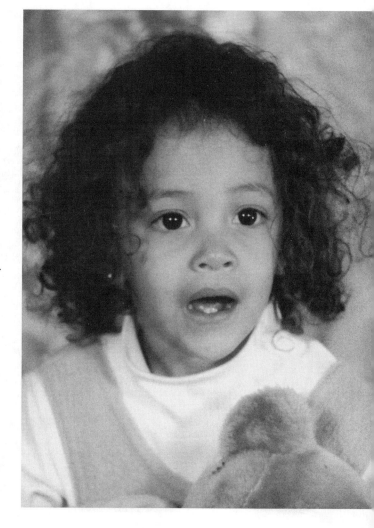

If Your Child Has Wavy Hair

The care of wavy hair is very similar to the care of curly hair, especially in infants and children up to two years old. Wavy hair does not require as much oil as other textures. Again, during the early years of your child's life, the most important task is shampooing with a product that is mild and gentle. Most baby shampoos are designed for those tender young scalps and new hair.

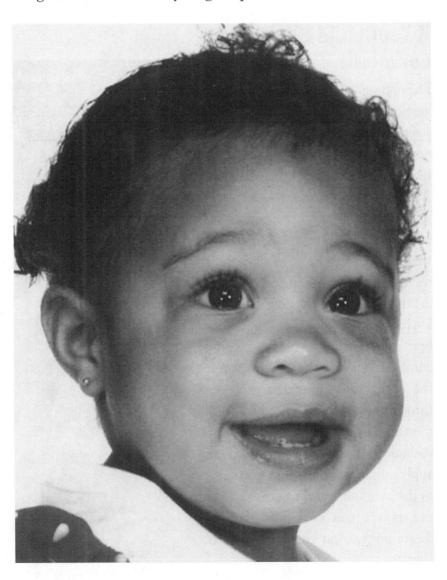

When you purchase combs and brushes, make sure they are child safe. Your child's brush should have soft bristles, and the comb should be plastic and not have sharp teeth. Infant combs and brushes are best for children under nine months. Test the teeth by putting them on your fingertips or on the back of your hand; if the teeth feel sharp to you, then the comb is too sharp for your child. It is important that you comb and brush your child's hair on a daily basis.

When children begin to sit up on their own, it is a good time to start using something to protect their eyes while shampooing their hair; baby shampoo visors work well for that purpose. Also, to make this time fun for your child and easier for you, purchase a shower attachment designed especially for babies. These items can be found where most infant merchandise is sold.

Your little one is growing up fast; let's see what's next.

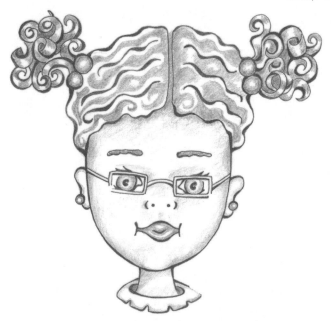

"I was so happy when my mom used a cream rinse on my hair. From that day on, if we didn't have cream rinse, I didn't get my hair washed. It made my hair soft, and it made the tangles go away easier. The comb with the big teeth helped, too."

Training Your Little Girl's Hair—Girls Two to Four Years Old

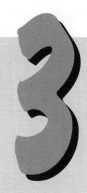

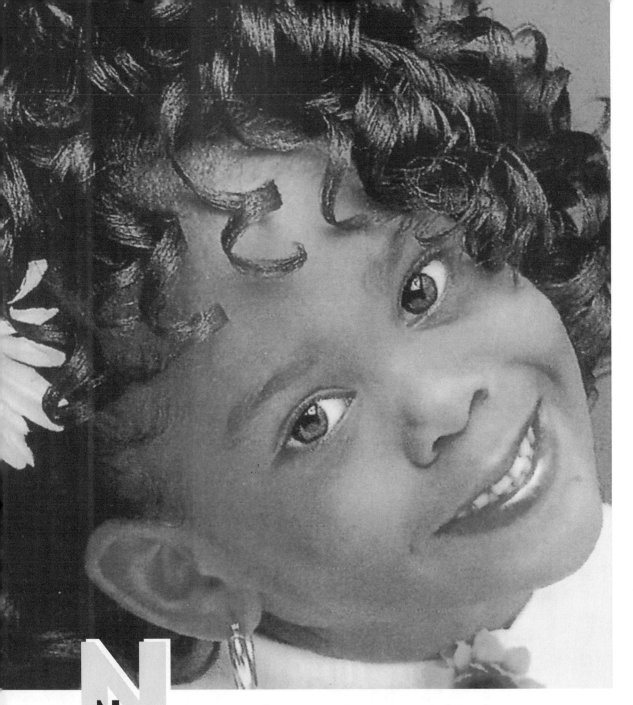

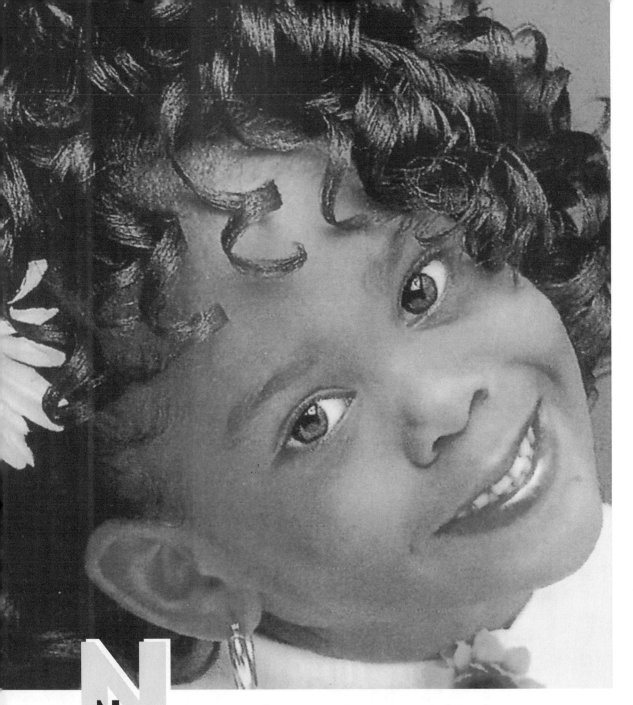**N**ow that your daughter is becoming more active, you have the choice of shampooing her hair in the shower, the bathtub, or the sink. If you shampoo in the tub or the sink, remember that eye protectors and a handheld shower head can make the process easier. You can purchase these items at most children's stores or discount stores.

For this age group you should continue to use baby shampoo, but you may alternate it with a mild children's shampoo. Most adult shampooss are designed for hair that has some kind of chemical in it and should be avoided. However, you can use products designed for natural (virgin) hair. Your child's shampoo should have a pH between 6 and 7, which is close to the pH of hair and skin. (Read the label or ask the salesperson to help you if you can't locate the information on the package.)

If you shampoo over the sink, start to comb the hair while it is dry, in the direction that you are going to shampoo it. You don't want to shampoo your child's hair upside down, but sometimes you may have to. If you do, just comb the hair first with a wide-tooth comb in that direction.

Shampoo the hair, making sure to use the tips of your fingers and not your nails. Remember to shampoo the hair in one direction for fewer tangles. Lather well and repeat if necessary. Rinse with warm water in the same direction you shampooed.

Apply the hair oil that is formulated for your child's hair texture. Since your child is still young, use a light oil made specifically for kids. As your child gets older, you can switch to a regular light oil made for adults. Your child's hair will tell you when to switch because the children's oil will no longer give the hair shine and pliability.

For painless combing, whether the hair is wet or dry, hold a portion of your child's hair at the root area somewhat tightly between your fingers. Be sure to have a nice grip on the hair so that when you begin to comb it, you are not pulling

MAKE IT FUN!

● ● ● ● ●

I found a handheld shower head that looks like a hippopotamus; it adds a bit of fun to this sometimes trying time.

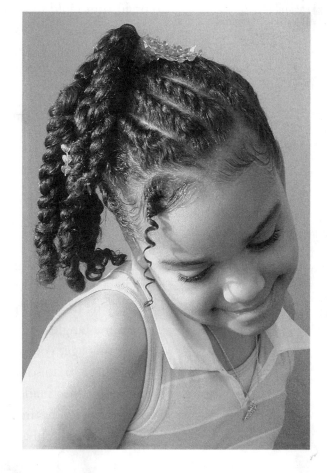

it from the scalp. Use a comb that matches the thickness of the hair. A good rule of thumb is to start off with a wide-tooth comb, in order to remove most of the tangles, and then work with a smaller-tooth comb if necessary. Holding a small portion of the hair, use the wide-tooth comb and start at the ends, working your way up toward the scalp. As you come closer to your closed hand or fingers, slowly open your hand and comb the hair toward you as you travel down to the scalp. Use combs that are hard plastic or hard rubber and brushes that are made of soft plastic or natural bristles. As your child's hair grows and the texture of it changes, you may need to change your combs and brushes to get the desired results.

Hair should be combed every day, but with today's busy schedules it doesn't always happen. That's not good. The safe alternative is to braid your child's hair into small braids, which allows the hair to stay neater longer. Always use safe plastic or cloth hair ornaments, and do not pull the hair too tightly. When you use hair ties with balls on the ends, be mindful of your child's hair type. If her hair is thick, medium, or coarse, you can use the larger versions, but if her hair is thin and fine, use the smaller ones.

If Your Child Has Kinky Hair

Using a mild shampoo on this hair texture is very important, particularly at this young age. As children get older, their hair will become drier. It is important to rinse kinky or excessively curly hair thoroughly because sometimes the shampoo can hide in between the curls, especially if the hair draws up tightly when it gets wet. When towel-drying the hair, squeeze it gently and don't tousle it, which can create more tangles.

At this age, your child's hair texture may start to change and you may have to do some experimenting. You should be able to find shampoo brushes made especially for children. These brushes help keep the hair going in one direction while cleansing the hair and scalp more thoroughly.

LESS STRESS

● ● ● ● ●

Work in sections when combing kinky hair. It makes the whole process go a lot more smoothly.

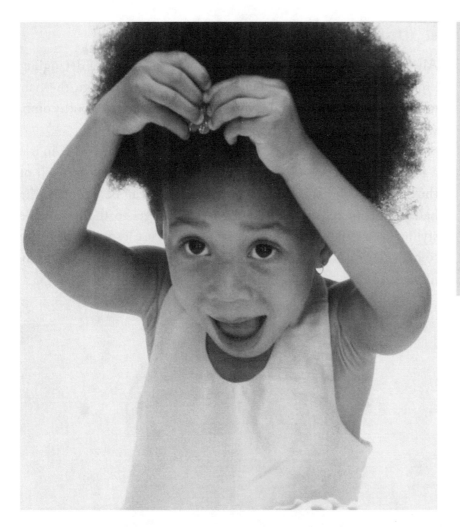

LESS STRESS

● ● ● ● ●

Cotton pillowcases are not the best for your child's hair, since cotton is a natural fiber and takes the moisture out of the hair. Buy a satin pillowcase instead.

After shampooing your child's hair, you should always apply a cream rinse or a detangler followed by hair cream, hair moisturizer, or hair oil. Sometimes these products can be used in combination and you will find they work even better. Although kinky hair does require more product, don't overload.

Kinky hair can be soft and kinky, medium and kinky, or coarse and kinky. The secret is to work with the hair and not against it. Work with small sections, give your child something to play with, and be gentle. It's better to work on damp hair and braid it as you go along; braiding allows the scalp to breathe.

LESS
STRESS
● ● ● ● ●

Wet hair combs far
more easily than
dry hair.

If Your Child Has Curly Hair

Always follow up a shampooing with a cream rinse or a detangling product designed for naturally curly hair. Comb through the hair using a wide-tooth comb and then switch to a medium-tooth comb, working in small sections from the ends to the root area.

If you would like your child's curls to stay in place, you can use a product that has some gel qualities to it. Don't use too much of these products for this age group because they can be drying to the hair. If you prefer, you can apply a light oil gel to the hair while styling it, especially around the hairline. Then use a soft bristle brush to help control those small hairs by making them lie down and stay in place.

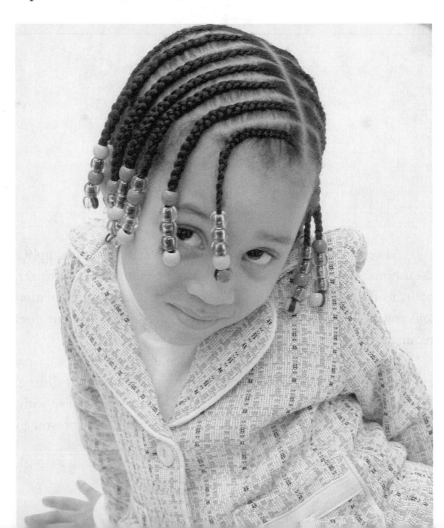

If Your Child Has Wavy Hair

After shampooing with a mild or children's shampoo, spray a detangler or a cream rinse onto your child's hair. Apply a very light hair cream or oil if your child's hair is dry, although dryness is uncommon for wavy hair textures. You can leave wavy hair loose, but braiding is better. Or if the hair is long enough, a ponytail is a pretty style.

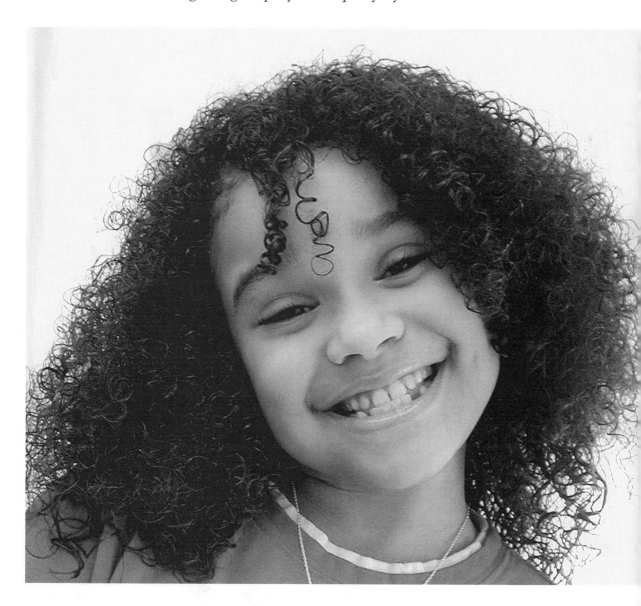

"My friend Kia has thick, curly hair, but it's kind of short. She said her mom cut it because she didn't know how to style it. So now the boys at school tease her. But I gave her some of my headbands and showed her how to make her hair look pretty. Yesterday, Joshua, a boy in her class, told her she was pretty. I think he likes her."

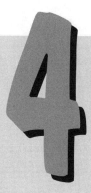

Time for Changes—Girls Four to Eight Years Old 4

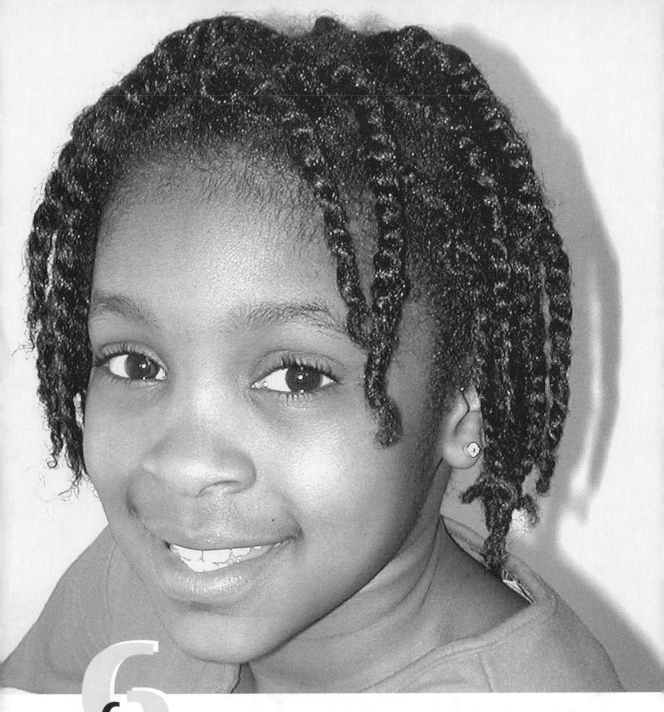

Growth, texture, and length are the direct results of genetics and how well you take care of your child's hair. Depending on the texture, the cuticle (the top layer of the hair) begins to lose moisture, becoming drier. Within the first year of your child's life, changes have begun. Beginning at three years old, your child's hair may look totally different from the hair he or she was born with. Believe it or not, this hair is going to change, too.

This second stage usually lasts until your child is eight or ten. The third stage is the growth of your child's permanent hair. In most cases, the true texture of your child's hair will have developed by the age of ten. And as your child's hair changes, so should the way you take care of it and the products you use on it.

When little girls reach the age of four, it may be time to try some new methods of hairstyling. The hair products you have been using should still work well on your little girl's hair, as should a wide-tooth comb.

Don't be too eager to use chemicals on her hair. Misusing chemicals on your daughter's fragile hair could cause permanent damage to the follicles, resulting in breakage or even bald spots. Hold out at least until your daughter is eight years old before applying any chemicals to her hair.

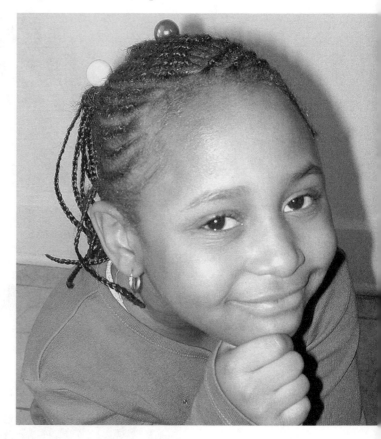

> **DON'T TAKE ANY CHANCES**
>
> ● ● ● ● ● ●
>
> Keep your daughter's hair in its natural state for as long as you can.

If Your Child Has Kinky Hair

Sometimes natural hairstyles can present a small problem for young girls because as they get older and go to school they want to wear their hair a different way. Kinky-looking hair isn't always very popular because of the misconception that style options are limited. To make matters worse, many little girls in this age group are teased about their hairstyle, but there are many pretty options for kinky hair.

If Your Child Has Curly Hair

Using the correct products is very important and will allow you to create the different hairstyles that young girls in this age group will start to want. Apply products, such as styling lotion or mousse, to damp hair, layer by layer. Start at the nape of the neck and rub the product in. If necessary, you can mix the product with a small amount of curl moisturizer. Then apply the product from the scalp to the ends, using your fingers to comb it through the hair. Move up to the next section of hair and continue the application process throughout the entire head.

Remember, the less you brush and comb curly hair, the better it will stay in place. Let the hair air-dry, if you can, and you will have a

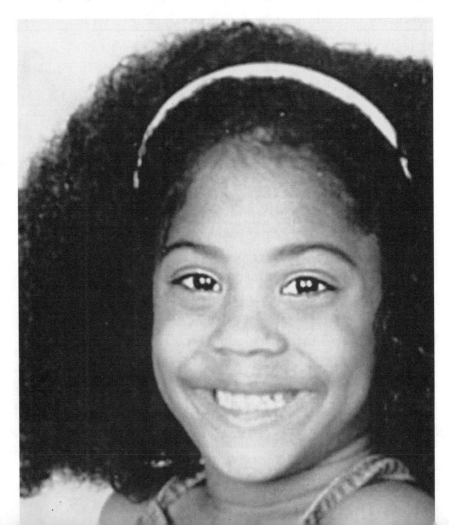

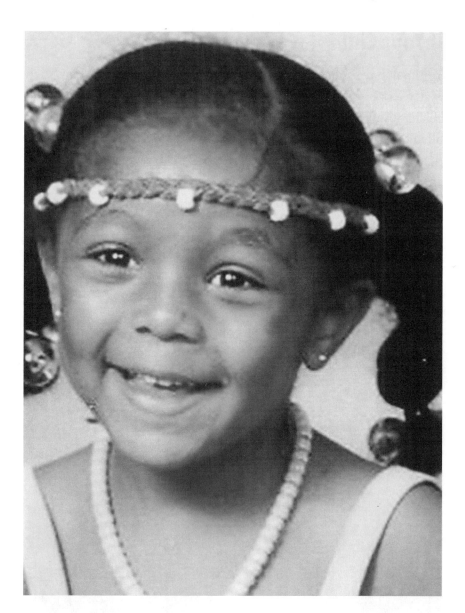

headful of pretty curls that aren't frizzy. Of course, this can only be done when you have the time and it's not cold outside.

Other options include using headbands, combs, and other hair accessories. There are so many pretty hair ornaments in stores today. Just make sure the ones you select do not pull out the hair when you remove them.

If Your Child Has Wavy Hair

You may have started to see some changes in your child's hair, such as dryness or oiliness. If your child's hair does become oily, it should be shampooed more often with a shampoo specifically designed for oily hair.

Astringents such as witch hazel or Sea Breeze are also good as an extra safety measure for oily scalps. To cleanse the scalp after shampooing, dilute the product with water (half astringent and half water) and apply it with a cotton swab; then use a light cream rinse made especially for oily hair and thoroughly rinse the hair.

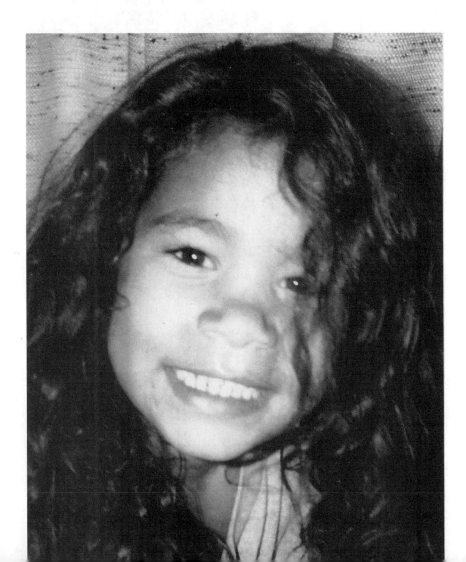

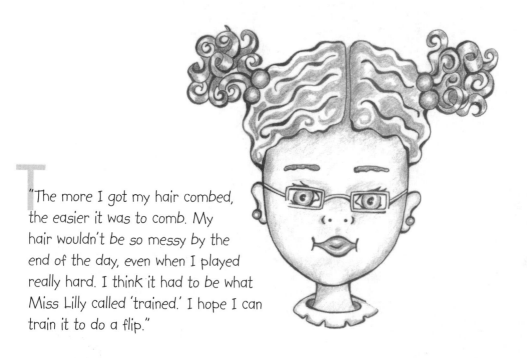

"The more I got my hair combed, the easier it was to comb. My hair wouldn't be so messy by the end of the day, even when I played really hard. I think it had to be what Miss Lilly called 'trained.' I hope I can train it to do a flip."

Growing Up—Girls Eight to Twelve Years Old

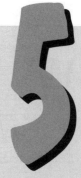

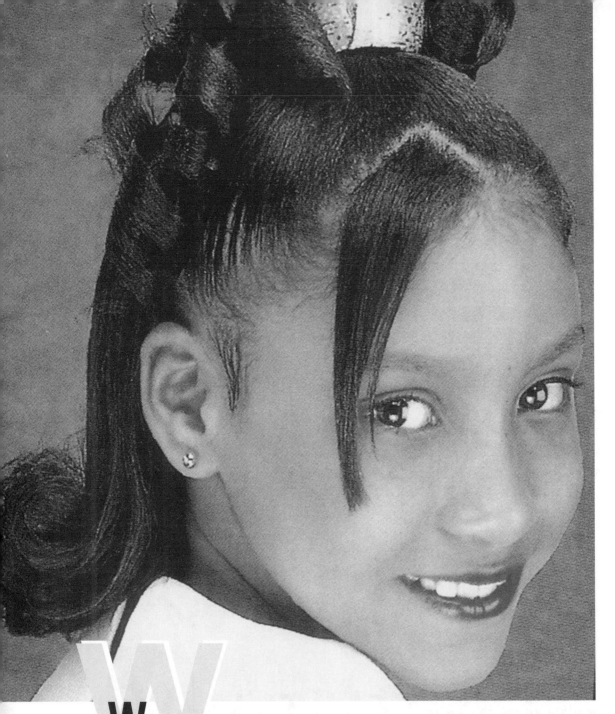

When it comes to hair, this period is a very exciting and sometimes trying time for girls. Everything about them is changing: their minds, bodies, and attitudes, and especially the way they see themselves. They begin to notice the hair of their friends, or their favorite singer, or a TV personality.

How their teacher's or their mom's hair looks might suddenly become interesting to them.

Many things influence how young girls want to look, especially when it comes to their hair. They may decide their hair looks better straight than curly, or short rather than long, or even in braids.

It is very important that you let your daughter know that whatever type of hair she has, she is a beautiful and special child. Even when your daughter knows that, she will still want her hair to look like her best friend's hair. Of course, her best friend has medium-length, red, curly hair and your daughter has long, black, wavy hair.

Tell your daughter that you can style her pretty hair in many different, special ways and that what is most important is keeping her hair healthy. Explain to her that when she gets older, if she still wants to wear her hair differently, she will be able to change it herself.

During this time, it would be a good idea to allow your daughter to select some really cool hair accessories and ornaments. There are headbands, bobby pins with rhinestones, star-shaped barrettes—lots of things she might like. Just make sure that the accessories are not too heavy and that when they are removed they will not pull her hair out. Ornaments that have fasteners made of metal often pull out strands of hair.

If Your Child Has Kinky Hair

Many girls between the ages of eight and twelve who have kinky hair are unhappy with their hair texture. Most often, it is because of teasing or because they want their hair to be long and silky. This is usually the group where I see hair that has been abused from trying to make it something that it is not. As early as possible, start taking good care of your daughter's kinky hair. You will have better results when she reaches her preteens.

Keep using a mild shampoo on your daughter's hair. If you find that the shampoo will not lather on dirty hair, try a cleansing or clarifying shampoo. Use it for the first soaping, then use the mild

DON'T TAKE ANY CHANCES

● ● ● ● ●

Most conditioners do not work well on virgin hair— hair that has no chemicals in it—so it's important to use a cream rinse followed by a detangler.

shampoo. There are also moisturizing shampoos on the market that work well on kinky hair.

The length of your daughter's hair helps you determine what you can and cannot do with it. If her hair is very short and very hard to comb or style, you may want to consider having it braided with extensions. Many times the constant pulling from the comb on dry kinky hair breaks it.

Giving your daughter's hair a break by having it braided with extensions is a great help. Twists, braids, and curls all work well because these styles can be worn for several days or more. If you decide to have your little girl's hair braided, keep her style youthful and age appropriate. Also, don't leave the braids in too long. You can read more about hair extensions in chapter 6.

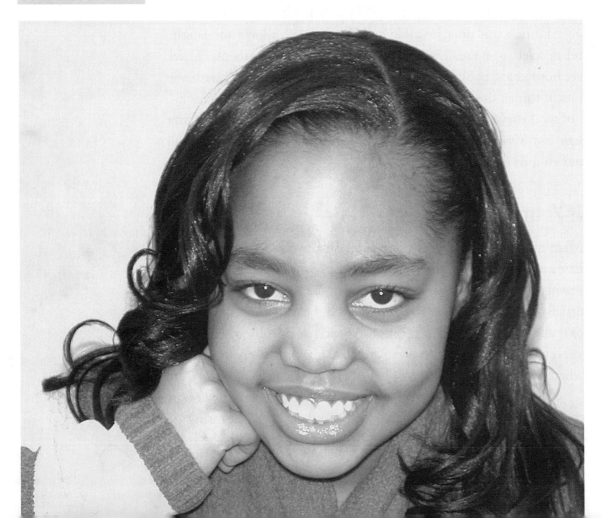

If your little one has medium-length to long hair, then you have a few more options. The resulting style all depends on the thickness, softness, or coarseness of the hair. Kinky hair can be kinky and soft, kinky and medium textured, or kinky and coarse. Kinky and soft hair really shrinks up when it gets wet. If you braid it for a couple of days, it will stretch and straighten out.

It's important to find the right hair oil or hairdressing cream. You can also use combinations. Try a product with a cream base and add a product that has an oil base. Together, the two ingredients give the hair just the right amount of oil and moisture.

Until your daughter was about ten, you might have been able to shampoo her hair, use a cream rinse, oil her hair and scalp, and control her hair with a good brush. Then one day, your daughter's hair started to get bushy. Now, to make matters worse, she wants to wear straight bangs and a ponytail. She may even ask you if she can wear her hair down sometimes. The solution to those requests is called warm combing, using a pressing comb to temporarily straighten the hair. Pressing your daughter's hair is discussed in chapter 7.

Another great alternative for kinky hair is cornrowing. Your daughter has the rest of her life to wear relaxed hair, if that is what she wants. Keep her hair clean, healthy, and braided for as long as you possibly can.

If your daughter wants to wear her hair natural and wild for a couple of days, let her. No harm done. At night, her hair should be either braided or on rollers. Teach her how to braid her hair and purchase a hair wrap so she can tie it up at night. Get your daughter involved with caring for her own hair; allow her to shampoo, and maybe even style, it herself.

After shampooing your daughter's hair, apply a cream rinse, followed by a detangler to help remove tangles from her natural hair. A moisturizing conditioner might also be helpful for your daughter's hair. Or apply a small amount of the moisturizing spray that is used on Jheri curls around the hairline. It makes kinky hair easier to comb, and it also nourishes the scalp.

LESS STRESS

Conditioners that contain olive oil, jojoba, coconut oil, or shea butter all work very well on kinky hair. But it's still important to use a cream rinse and a detangler every time you wash the hair.

Remember to keep your daughter's hair going in the same direction. Apply a detangler and a small amount of moisturizing spray. Part a small section of hair in the nape area or wherever you may want to start braiding. By now you should be a pro at detangling with your wide-tooth comb, starting at the ends and moving toward the scalp. Finally, if the hair and scalp look and feel dry, apply some oil to both areas. Once you have combed out a section of hair, you should always braid or twist it before you move on to the next section. There's more on braiding in chapter 6.

If Your Child Has Curly Hair

For some little girls in this age group, curly hair can also be discouraging. It all depends on how tight the curls are, how thick the hair is, and how long the hair is. Many times we don't know how to control thick, curly hair, and your daughter has become dissatisfied with the way her hair looks. She wants her hair to be straight, worried that her thick, curly hair makes her look funny.

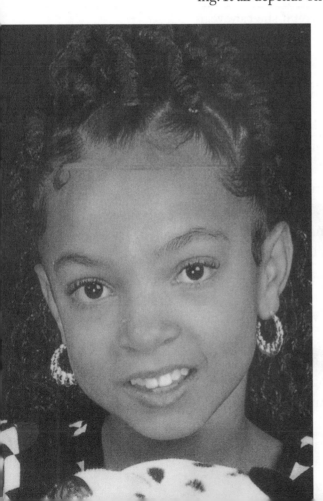

When you shampoo curly hair, keep your hands on the scalp and work underneath the hair. Make sure you have a rich, full lather, otherwise you are not getting the shampoo into those curves and coils.

Rinse your daughter's hair thoroughly, always keeping it flowing in the same direction. With thick, curly hair especially, you should rinse until you see the water running clear. Apply a cream rinse, followed by a detangler. Rinse well and gently squeeze the excess water out of the hair.

Put some moisturizing conditioner into your daughter's hair. Let it sit in the hair, then comb it through using a wide-tooth comb. The thicker the hair, the longer it should be conditioned, up to twenty minutes. If you prefer, you can seat your daughter under a hooded dryer with a plastic cap on her head. Then do a final rinse and gently towel-dry the hair in the same direction that it was shampooed. Finally, apply a leave-in conditioner, and then, working in small sections, comb the hair using a wide-tooth comb.

It is very important to do all these steps with the hair flowing in the same direction, because it makes it much easier to comb and creates less tangling and matting.

While curly hair is still damp, you should apply curl-control products. I list some in the back of this book. Saturate the hair with the product, using your fingers to massage it in, then comb through. The less you do to your daughter's curly hair, the better it will look.

If you have gotten to the point where this doesn't work and the hair is too unruly and wild, you might want to use a relaxer or a texturizer to control the curl. Chapter 10 tells you how to tame curly hair with a texturizer. If used properly, relaxers can be gentle and safe and will work like magic. Try to wait until your daughter is at least ten before you take this step.

DO YOUR RESEARCH

Moisturizers are essential for curly hair. Look for ingredients like amino acids, glycerine, aloe vera, and panthenol. Always read the labels, and stay away from products that contain large amounts of alcohol.

If Your Child Has Wavy Hair

By this time, your child's hair texture has pretty much become what it is going to be. It might become a little straighter, wavier, or thicker, but unlike when your daughter was an infant, the texture is not going to change drastically.

If your daughter's hair is soft, most likely it is going to stay soft. Continue to use a mild shampoo on her hair. You don't want to use a shampoo that will strip the natural oils from her hair. If her hair is fine and thin, you may be tempted to use a product that says it will add volume. Many of those types of products have ingredients that can dry out the hair, causing breakage. If her hair is thick, you can use a moisturizing conditioner. To keep the hair in place, use a moisturizing mousse, styling lotion, or light gel.

You can also use products that contain natural ingredients such as rosemary, basil, and chamomile. If you live in an area where there is a natural foods store, check out some of the hair care products.

If your daughter wants a change, think about getting her hair cut into a one-length style, like a bob, or letting her have bangs. A bob will help her hair stay in place and appear thicker. These kinds of changes also give her the ability to style her own hair because now it's more manageable. Your daughter may even become a trendsetter among her friends. Also, around the age of ten, many girls want to do their own hair, and that's a good thing. Show them what to do and let them go for it. Just don't let them try to cut their own hair or put any heat to it. I have seen hair burned from using Mom's curling irons, and I've seen a lot of short, short bangs. The good news is, it's only hair and it will grow back. If you are at that point where your daughter wants a little more variety, there are many options coming up.

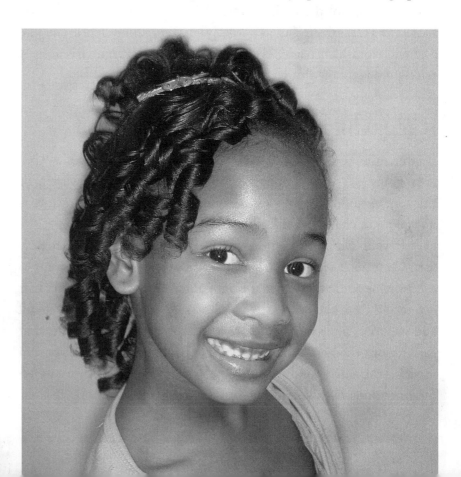

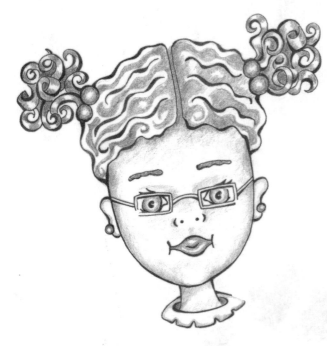

"Braiding is safe, and you can make so many different styles. Mom says it's healthy for my hair, too. I really like to put pretty beads on the ends of my hair, and I get to pick the ones I like; but I don't like it when my braids are too tight. It makes little bumps come up on my scalp."

Braiding Your Daughter's Hair

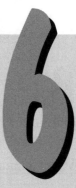

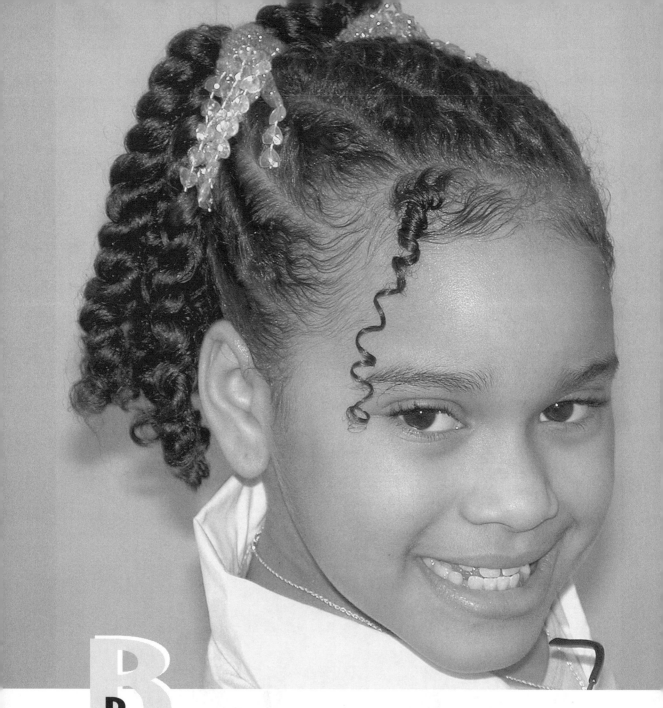

By far, braids are one of the healthiest hairstyles for your little one. Braiding, when done properly, gives the hair control and allows the scalp to breathe.

The most important factor when braiding is not to make the braids too tight. When braids are too tight, they pull the scalp, especially around the hairline. You

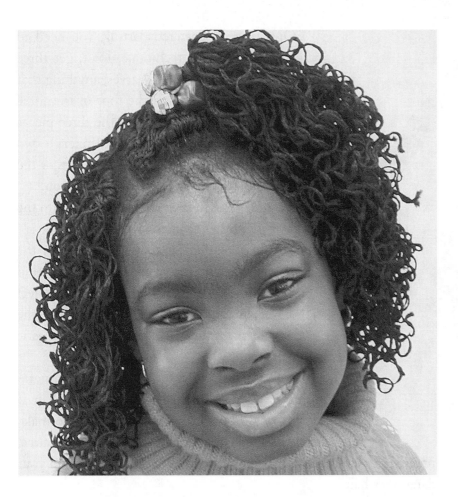

may not see it right away, but the stress will soon begin to show. In some cases, when girls start to get their hair relaxed after having worn braids for a while, the edges of their hair break off or become very thin. Be aware of this when your daughter gets her hair braided.

Single Braids

This is the simplest and easiest form of braiding. Begin by making clean partings in the hair. This is easy to do with the tip of a rattail comb (a small comb with a skinny pointed handle), or you can use the teeth of a regular comb. The best method to use will depend on the thickness and length of your daughter's hair.

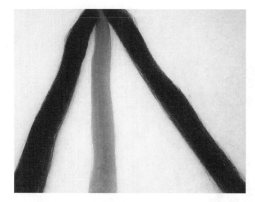

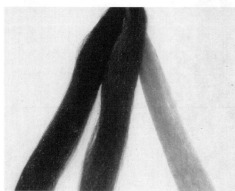

Once you've mastered parting, you need to work on the braiding technique. First, get three pieces of thick yarn or three scarves; anything that you can easily tie. Next, tie the tops of the three pieces together in a knot. Spread the three pieces between your index and middle fingers—two pieces in the right hand and one in the left, or the combination that is most comfortable for you.

Now take the first strand and cross it into the middle of the other two strands. Take the outside strand from the other hand and cross it over the middle strand. Continue crossing the right strand over the middle strand, then crossing the left strand over the middle strand. When you reach the ends, secure the braid with a safe cloth or plastic hair ornament.

Now try this with your daughter's hair, starting off with medium-size sections. If her hair is short it might be a little harder to grasp, so make smaller-size sections and then practice, practice, practice. It should take you about a day to learn how to braid your daughter's hair.

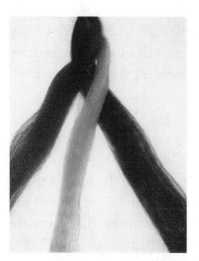

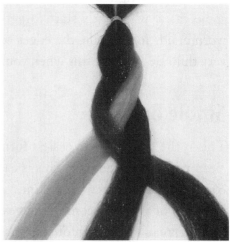

Cornrowing

This method of braiding is an extension of regular single braiding. Once you and your daughter have decided what cornrowed hairstyle she prefers, you can begin by making small, long, narrow sections in the direction that you want the braids to go. When cornrowing, the sections of hair should be long and thin, about one quarter inch to one inch wide.

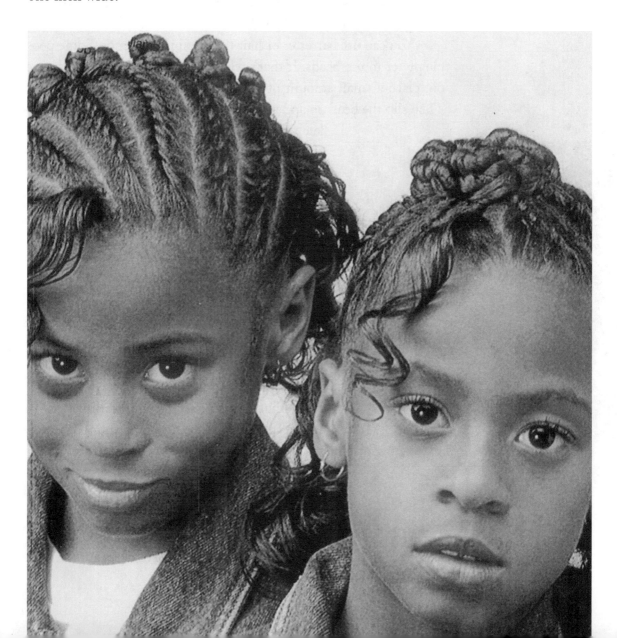

Take three small subsections from the front of the hair, and place your fingers underneath so that the braid forms on top of the hair. Start the same movement as in single braiding, but as you braid downward, grab hair and join it with the hair that you are moving from left to right. This may sound confusing, but with practice it becomes simple. Continue taking the right strand and the left strand as in single braiding, picking up hair from underneath and joining it with the strands that are forming the braid. Continue this motion until you get to the end of the hair.

You can use barrettes or hair ties to finish the ends. Some people prefer to use beads. If that's what you and your daughter decide on, place a small amount of gel on the end of the braided strand. Then slip the bead on and wrap a small rubber band over the end to keep the bead in the hair; or you can tie yarn on the end of the braid and thread the beads into the hair. If your daughter's hair is fine and thin, do not put too many beads onto one strand because the weight of the beads could actually weaken her hair.

French Braiding

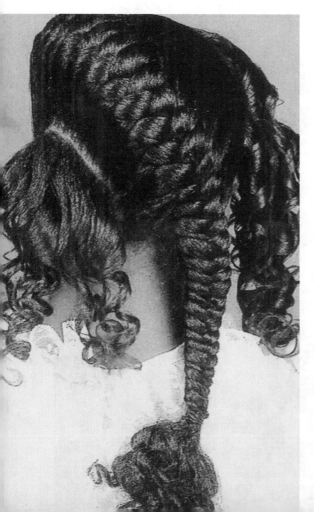

With this style of braiding, your daughter's hair must be fairly long and the sections are usually on the larger side. You have the option of braiding either over or under, but there are specific rules that determine the actual direction in which you braid. To begin, comb your daughter's hair back, going straight down the center of her head. Now make three parted sections starting at the top of the head. If you want the braid to be inside the hair, your fingers will be on top of the strands; if you want the braid to be on the outside, your fingers should be underneath the hair.

Just as you would do in cornrowing, begin the French braiding process as if you are making a single braid. As you braid, pick up hair from both sides and join that hair with the initial section. This movement will cause you to travel down the head until you come to the ends. Since you are using large sections of hair, this method can be a little more difficult. As with many of these techniques, you will need practice, but it's really a very pretty hairstyle for girls with medium-length and long hair.

Extensions

Extensions are added hair to make the natural hair look fuller and longer. Depending on the style, extensions can be worn from three weeks to three months, but they must be taken care of properly. If you want your little girl to wear braids for an extended period of time, this would be the best method.

There are special products on the market to help maintain braids. Shampoo and condition your daughter's hair at least every two weeks, and spray it with braid moisturizer as needed. This will keep her hair and scalp from drying out.

To keep your daughter's style fresh, tie her hair up at night with a satin scarf. In most African American neighborhoods there is someone who knows how to do cornrows using extensions, or you can always go to a professional hairstylist who braids.

Braided extensions should not be left in the hair too long; the time varies depending on the style. Usually, if the braids are small, they can be worn for a longer period of time, but never more than eight weeks. If your daughter's hair is braided repeatedly over a year's time, you can expect three to six inches of new growth.

Braids must be shampooed. For best results, take a stocking cap or a hairnet and place it over your daughter's braids before you shampoo. Using a mild or special braid shampoo, gently massage her hair and scalp, and then rinse until the water runs clear. Apply conditioner and rinse again. Next, spray her hair with a

LESS STRESS

● ● ● ● ●

Many braid professionals suggest that synthetic hair be used on young girls because it requires less maintenance than human hair extensions.

braid spray and sit your daughter under a hood dryer; this will keep the braids nice and soft. Finally, lightly oil your daughter's scalp, but be careful not to use too much oil because it may cause the extensions to loosen and slip off.

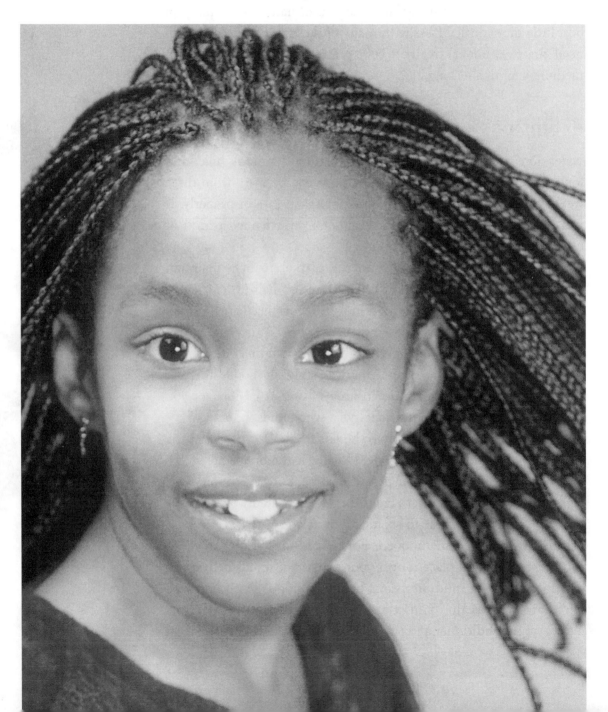

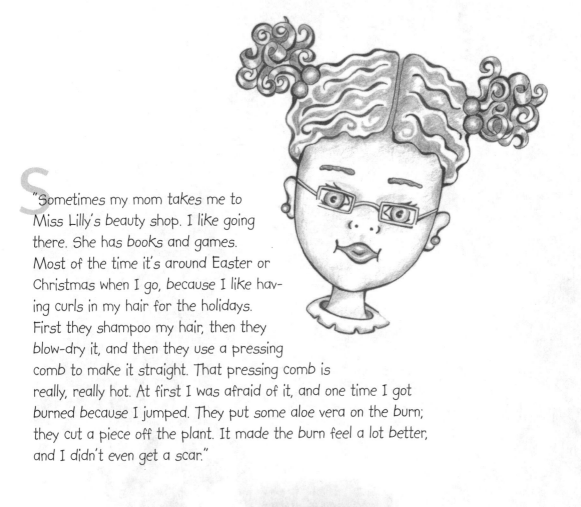

"Sometimes my mom takes me to Miss Lilly's beauty shop. I like going there. She has *books* and games. Most of the time it's around Easter or Christmas when I go, because I like having curls in my hair for the holidays. First they shampoo my hair, then they blow-dry it, and then they use a pressing comb to make it straight. That pressing comb is really, really hot. At first I was afraid of it, and one time I got burned because I jumped. They put some aloe vera on the burn; they cut a piece off the plant. It made the burn feel a lot better, and I didn't even get a scar."

Pressing Your Daughter's Hair

7

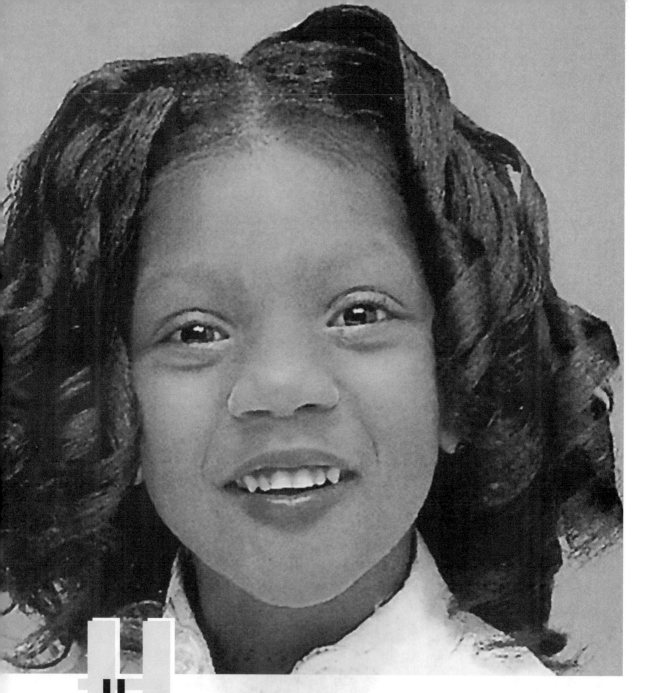

Hair pressing is an African American technique that dates as far back as the 1870s. It is a method for making the hair temporarily straight; as long as the hair doesn't get wet or isn't exposed to excessive humidity, it will stay straight. Years ago you could smell and see your hair frying, but it turned out pretty and shiny; and believe it or not, it was healthy, too.

Today's methods of hair pressing are not quite like they were in the old days. We don't use as much oil, or "grease," as it was called back then, and the look is much more natural.

For young ladies between the ages of eight and twelve, the main purpose of hair pressing is to make the hair more manageable and prettier.

Pressing is recommended if your daughter's hair has a tight curl and you want her hair to be easier to comb. Warm combing, however, is a better option for at-home styling, especially if your daughter is under the age of eight. That means the pressing comb is not as hot as it would be if you were trying to give what's called a hard press, which is better for older girls or adults with kinky hair.

Step 1: Purchasing Your Pressing Tools

Begin by selecting a pressing comb. Pressing combs can have large, medium, or small teeth, but I prefer the medium- and small-toothed ones. Some pressing combs are designed with curved teeth, some have straight teeth—both will do the job.

These types of pressing combs must be heated up by placing them on top of fire or by putting them into a stove that's especially designed for curling irons, flat irons, and pressing combs. If you are anxious about pressing in general, try using an electric pressing comb. They usually have a temperature control, so they don't get as hot, and they are easier to use.

> **LESS STRESS**
>
> If you're worried about pressing your daughter's hair, ask someone who's knowledgeable to give you a lesson.

Step 2: Shampooing and Drying

Begin by shampooing your daughter's hair as usual. Once you have shampooed and towel-dried her hair, apply a cream rinse or a leave-in detangler. Comb it through her hair, starting at the ends, and make six or seven braids.

LESS STRESS

● ● ● ● ● ●

In some cases, if you use a blow-dryer, you can actually skip the whole pressing process.

If you have a hood dryer, seat your daughter under it. The drying time will depend on the length and thickness of her hair. While she is under the dryer, feel her hair. As it becomes dry, undo your daughter's braids, loosening them so that the heat can penetrate into her hair. You don't want the hair to become tangled, so the less movement of the hair, the better.

You can also use a blow-dryer with a comb attachment. Blow-drying involves more work on your part and more stamina on the child's part, but this method dries and straightens the hair at the same time.

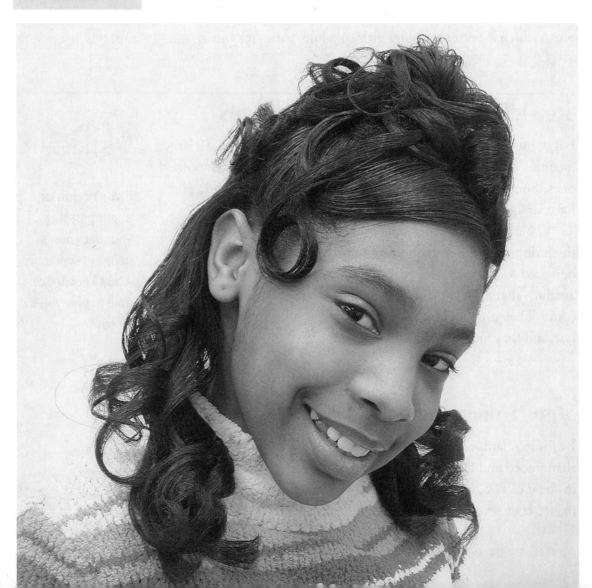

If you choose to use a blow-dryer, take the six or seven braids you made and dry each section one at a time. Start slowly at the ends and gently work your way to the scalp. The hair must be totally dry before you can press it. After you have dried each section, pin or twist it up out of your way.

Step 3: It's Time to Press

If you are using an electric pressing comb, it should be preheated on a medium setting. Once you begin, if you need more heat, you can turn the temperature up some. You should also have a small white cloth or towel nearby. If the towel turns brown when you touch it with the pressing comb, then the comb is too hot to put into your daughter's hair. Wait a minute and test the pressing comb again to see if it's cooled down enough to use on her hair.

Now, let's start pressing! First, apply a small amount of pressing oil to your daughter's hair (but not to her scalp, which could cause her scalp to burn). Pressing oil is a little heavier than other oils because it is formulated to enhance the pressing method, which is heat and pressure being applied simultaneously to achieve silky-straight hair. There are also various pressing solutions on the market that help achieve good results. Most are sprays, and they should be applied to clean, wet hair before it is dried and pressed.

The secret of a good pressing is to use the back or top of the pressing comb when you put the comb into the hair. First, take a small section of hair, about one by two inches. You have to use small sections to get the hair straight.

Take the heated pressing comb, test it, and simply comb it through the section of hair to remove the tangles. This will be your first run through the hair. Now run the comb through your daughter's hair again, this time slowly. As you comb, turn the pressing comb so that the back of it is actually touching and pressing her hair. Go through this same section a few more times until it looks the way

LESS STRESS

○ ○ ○ ○ ○

Pinning, braiding, and twisting may seem time-consuming, but the more you do it, the quicker and easier it gets.

you want it to. You may need to give the pressing comb some more heat if you are using one that must be warmed up in a stove. Repeat this process throughout the entire head, section by section, step by step.

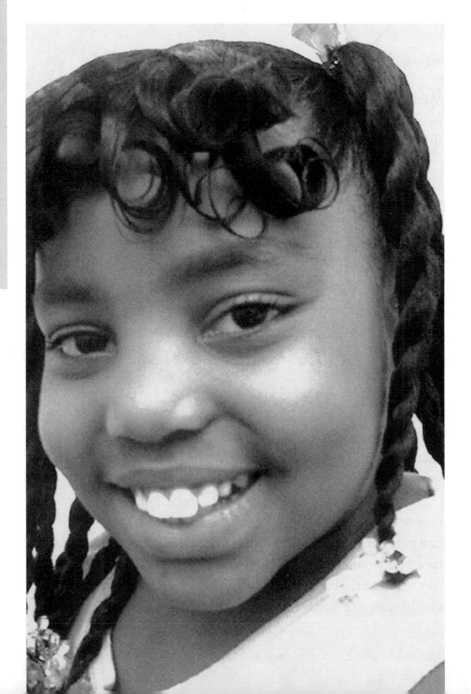

When pressing around the hairline, or edges, hold the hair very taut, but gently, with the tips of your fingers. Blow as you place the pressing comb to your daughter's hair. Most little ones do not like to get their hair pressed because they are afraid of the heat and of the possibility of being burned. Let your daughter blow on the pressing comb before you put it into her hair to cool it, or comb it through your own hair first to show her that it doesn't hurt.

Once your daughter's hair is pressed all over, you can finish by braiding it, putting it into ponytails, twisting it, or making bangs. If pressing feels like too much work, there are other methods of straightening the hair.

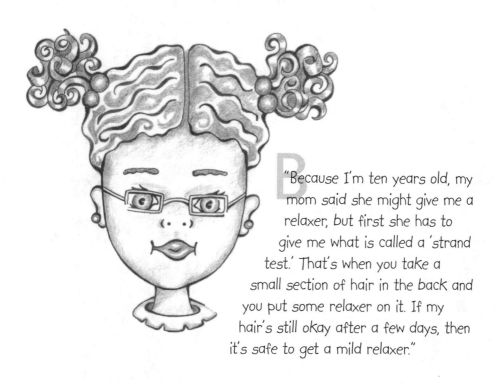

"Because I'm ten years old, my mom said she might give me a relaxer, but first she has to give me what is called a 'strand test.' That's when you take a small section of hair in the back and you put some relaxer on it. If my hair's still okay after a few days, then it's safe to get a mild relaxer."

Preparing Your Chemical Straightener or Relaxer

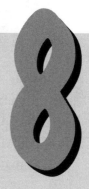

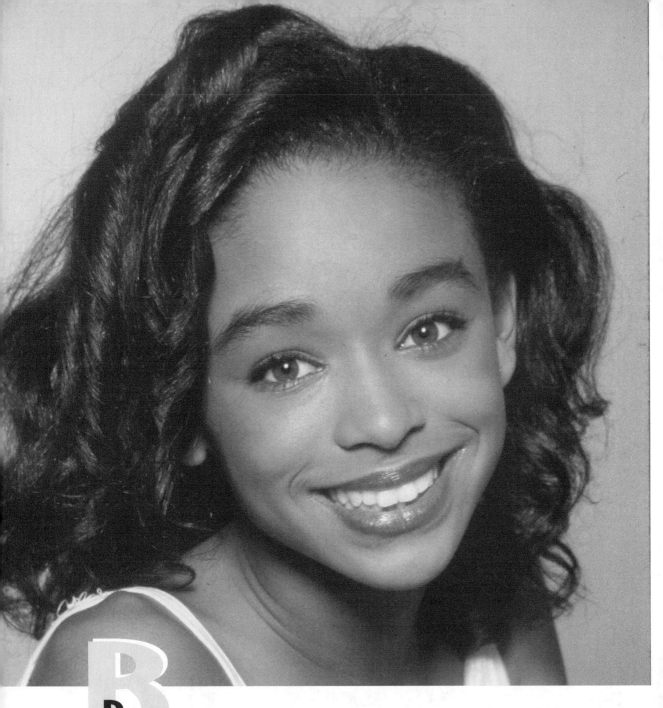

Before we go through the steps to relax your daughter's hair, it is important to devote a chapter to preparation. You should be knowledgeable about these products or you can cause serious damage to your child's hair and scalp.

Fortunately, many African American beauty companies have put a lot of time and money into research and development to provide us with quality products. There are some excellent relaxers on the market today for our little girls, but you still must know what to do with the product and how to take care of their hair.

Hair can be very tricky; it can look one way and act another. The key is still to know the texture of your daughter's hair. Just because your daughter's cousin had a relaxer doesn't mean that your daughter should have that same relaxer, or any relaxer at all.

Manufacturers recommend doing a strand test before you apply relaxer to the entire head. When you do a strand test, you apply the relaxer to a small area of the hair to see what kind of reaction your child's hair will have. If the hair has a negative reaction such as breakage, or if the scalp develops a rash or a burn, it is advised not to give your child a relaxer. Be patient and wait a little while. In most cases, as your daughter grows, her reaction to relaxers will change.

Relaxers come in different strengths, which is the relaxer's ability to straighten the hair. Some relaxers are too strong for your daughter's hair type, and some relaxers will do nothing at all. How you apply the relaxer may also give you some control over its straightening power. I will explain how in the next chapter.

Wait until your daughter is about ten years old before you give her a relaxer. If her hair is much too hard to handle and you must relax it, eight is as early as I would suggest that you apply chemicals to her hair.

Kiddie relaxers are designed to be less irritating to the scalp. When you purchase a kiddie relaxer kit, all of the necessary products are included. You will find pre-relaxer protector cream, relaxer cream, activator, neutralizing shampoo, conditioner, hair oil, setting lotion, and plastic gloves. Relaxer kits also contain step-by-step instructions, and some may even include a videotape. The only thing not included in a relaxer kit is a rattail comb.

It is important that you have a timer or a clock nearby so that you can keep track of how long the relaxer has been in your daughter's hair. You don't want to leave the relaxer in too long. Relaxers

DON'T TAKE ANY CHANCES

● ● ● ● ●

I have heard horror stories about little girls who were just three and four years old when someone put a "kiddie relaxer" into their hair. The little girls' scalps were burned and their hair broke off. As young adults, they continue to have serious problems with hair loss.

LESS
STRESS

● ● ● ● ● ●

A rattail comb is the best tool for applying a relaxer. If you prefer, you may apply it with an application brush, which will also be useful when it's time to give your daughter a touch-up.

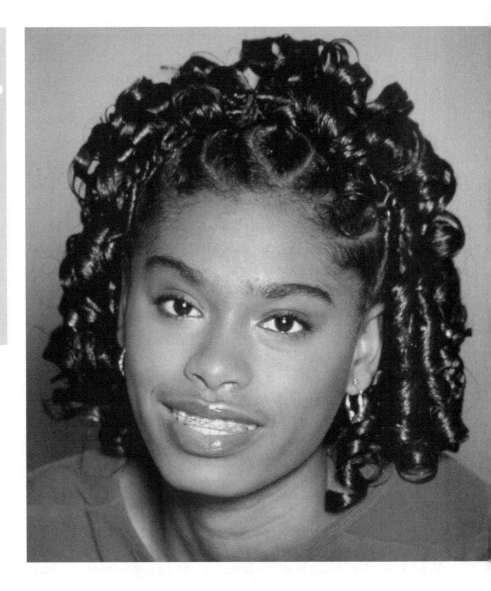

come in different strengths: mild for soft hair, regular for medium-textured hair, and super for very coarse, stubborn, or kinky hair. Some relaxer kits may have different descriptions for the specific strength that you will need for your daughter's hair texture. If you purchase your kit in a beauty-supply store as opposed to a super-market or a drugstore, you can find an informed salesperson to help you select the appropriate product.

Once you are ready to begin, thoroughly read the manufacturer's instructions and make sure you understand them. Unlike traditional relaxers that have a lye base, kiddie relaxers have a calcium, potassium, or mild chemical base. They also contain a liquid or cream solution usually referred to as activator. The activator is very important because it makes the relaxer work by giving it straightening power.

If your little girl has kinky but soft hair, and you just want to loosen her natural curl pattern, use a mild relaxer formula. With some of the kiddie kits, the manufacturers instruct you on how to use less activator, such as three-quarters of it instead of the whole bottle, in order to lessen the strength of the relaxer.

Some people are against putting chemical relaxers into a young girl's hair. You are using chemicals, so there is a risk of damaging the hair and skin, among other potential problems. If you take the time to read and understand the instructions, relaxers can be applied and worn safely. In close to thirty years of relaxing hair, I haven't had a client develop any health problems from relaxed hair. The ultimate decision is yours. You do not want to start a chemical process too early, but only you and your little girl know what you have been going through when it comes to caring for her hair.

Remember, you always have a choice when it comes to how you want your child's hair to look. Most of us want our children to have hair that is easy to comb and maintain. If you are in an area where you cannot find a good professional hairstylist and if you cannot relax your daughter's hair yourself, then it may be best for her to wear it in a natural style. It's the hair she was born with, and it's wonderful.

As African Americans, we are so lucky because we have so many hairstyle choices. Braids, afros, twists, locks, or straight hair can all be beautiful when we take care of them. If you still want to relax your daughter's hair, read on.

DON'T TAKE ANY CHANCES

● ● ● ● ●

Never use a super-strength relaxer unless you are 100 percent sure your daughter's hair needs it and you know exactly what you are doing.

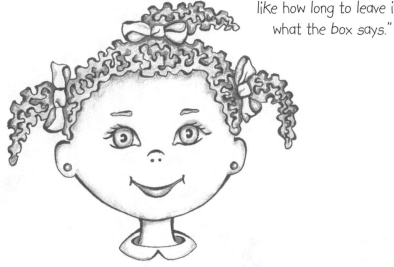

"My mom says I'm not old enough to have a relaxer. She says that my hair isn't ready. If she does give me one when I'm Berna's age, there's a lot she has to think about, like how long to leave it on and what the box says."

Relaxing Kinky Hair

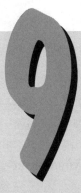

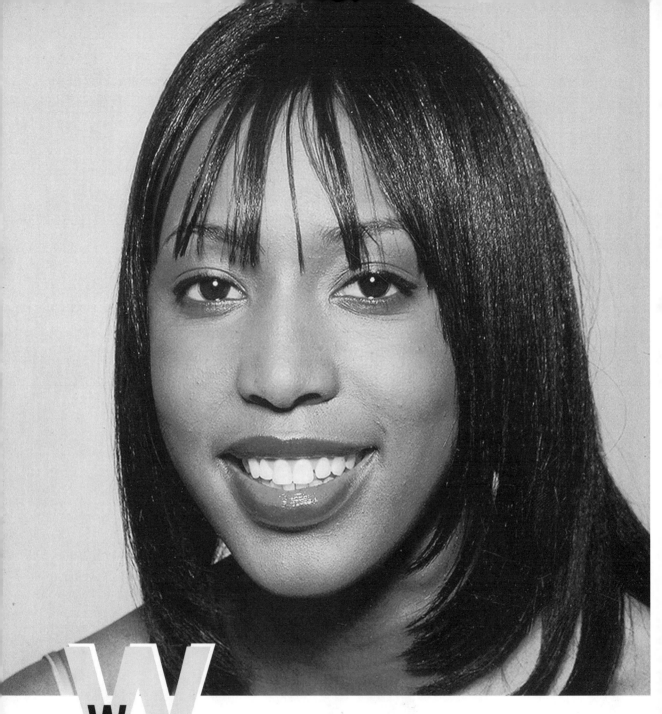

With your first chemical relaxer application, do not try to get the hair super straight. This could do more harm than good. Instead, your goal is to make the hair more manageable and easier to comb. If you don't get your daughter's hair as straight as you want it the first time, you will have many more opportunities to accomplish this.

The Examination

After reading the manufacturer's instructions, look at your daughter's hair and scalp. Examine it for any cuts, sores, or bruises. If you see any, you may have to wait until her scalp is healed. Ask your daughter if she has been scratching her head. If so, you can either wait twenty-four to forty-eight hours or coat the scalp with the base/protector cream.

Protection Is a Plus

Inside the relaxer kit, you will find the products that you need. Most kits will include a pre-relaxer protective cream.

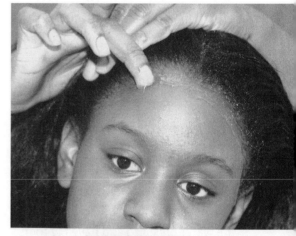

First, part your daughter's hair into four jumbo sections. Part going down the center and across the head from ear to ear, then twist and secure each section with a hair clip. Take the protective cream and apply it generously all around your daughter's hairline. You want to see it on the skin and on the tops and backs of the ears.

Next, section by section, part the hair into quarter-inch to half-inch sections and apply the cream to the scalp, but not too heavily. This cream acts as a covering for the skin and the scalp; it's okay if some of it gets onto the hair. The protective cream also stops the relaxer from penetrating the hair too quickly, which can be good if the hair is thick and you need more time to apply the relaxer.

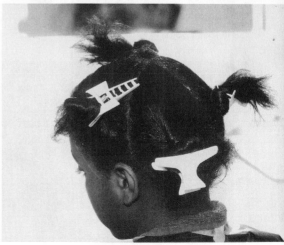

Do not rake the comb against the scalp at any time while parting or combing the hair into place. Gently, use the thin tip of a rattail comb to make the sections so that you will not have to touch the scalp too much. Before you

I had to rinse out my goddaughter's hair in the yard using a garden hose because there was no water pressure in the house. Her hair was so long and thick that I needed extra pressure to remove the relaxer from her hair and scalp. Talk about hard work! The water was cold and went everywhere. It's a good thing it was hot outside. I rinsed out most of the relaxer in the yard and then took my goddaughter inside the house, where I was able to finish rinsing out the rest of the relaxer.

This was in the very early days of my career as a hairdresser, and it could have turned out to be a real disaster. Needless to say, I don't rinse hair outside anymore, and I make sure to test the water pressure and have my tools ready before I use any chemicals.

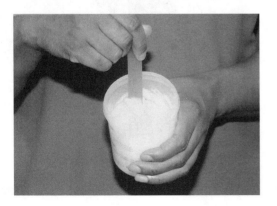

begin the application, it is very important to make sure you have shampoo and conditioner nearby. Also, set out two or three towels: one to drape around your daughter's shoulders (if you're not using a cape), one to cover her face, and one to dry her hair. You may even want something to plug her ears.

Mixing the Relaxer

Now you are ready to combine the relaxer cream and the activator, which are packaged separately inside the relaxer kit. Mix the two ingredients thoroughly using the wooden spatula that comes in the kit or something plastic. Never use metal to mix these two chemicals. Let the mixed relaxer sit for a few minutes while you put on your plastic gloves, also included in the kit.

Before you begin the relaxer application, check and make sure your water source has good water pressure. Decide exactly where you are going to rinse your daughter's hair and make sure that you have the area set up with the necessary tools. Your daughter should be sitting up high enough so that her head can reach the water. Also, decide if she will be leaning forward, with her head over the sink, or if you will be rinsing her hair as she lies backward into the sink. (Your beauty-supply store should have a special shampoo hose or nozzle.) Sometimes you have to start rinsing the hair quickly and you don't want any obstacles when the time comes.

Beginning the Application Process

Before you begin the application, drape a towel or a shampoo cape around your daughter's shoulders. With gloved hands, start to apply the relaxer to the crown of your daughter's head, beginning at either the right or the left back section. Take a quarter-inch to a half-inch section, depending on the thickness and coarseness of her hair, and begin applying the relaxer on the top layer of that section, about an inch away from the scalp.

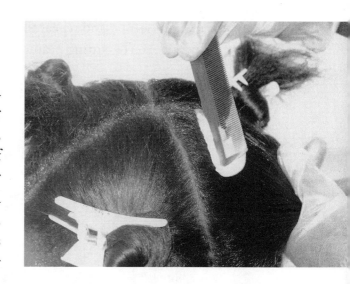

Apply it to the length of the hair, stopping about half an inch from the ends. Then lift up the section and apply the relaxer underneath, letting the hair fall forward. Take another small section, and working your way down, apply the relaxer to the top of the section and then underneath. Let that hair fall forward on top of the last section you did.

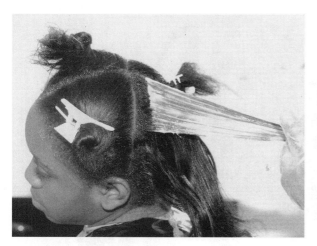 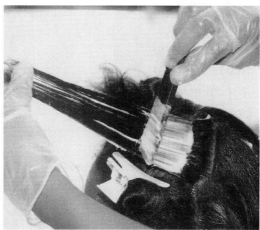

Continue to work your way down until you come to the last section at the nape of the neck. Then move on to the next back section and repeat the same steps. You should apply the relaxer as if you're putting peanut butter on a slice of bread.

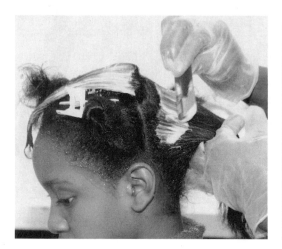 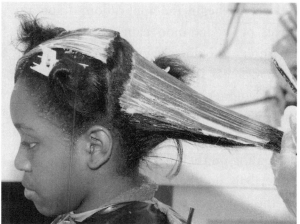

After you have finished the application to the back of the head, move to the front. Starting at the middle section of the head, and working your way toward the ear, apply the relaxer in the same manner. Move to the opposite side and repeat the same steps.

RELAX:
Be Careful

If at any time you drop relaxer onto your daughter's face, neck, or skin, wipe it off immediately. This is why you should always have a clean towel nearby when you're giving a relaxer.

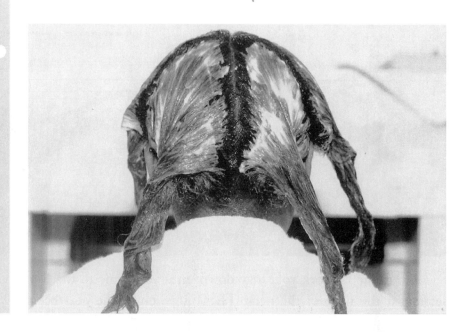

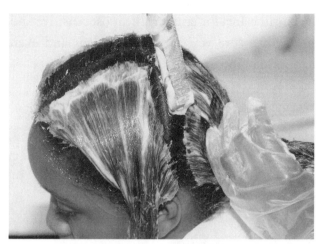
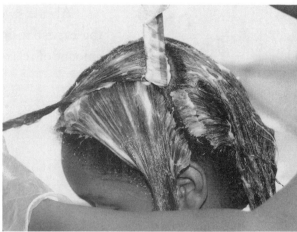

Applying the Relaxer Near the Scalp

Now you are ready to go back to the area where you started. Apply the relaxer a quarter-inch away from the scalp, instead of one inch from the scalp as you did the first time. Before you begin this final application, ask your daughter how she's feeling. If she is comfortable, continue to apply the relaxer closer to the scalp, maintaining the quarter-inch margin. The relaxer is applied this way because of the heat generated by our body: the hair closest to the scalp takes less time to straighten. Also, to protect the roots, we don't want the relaxer to remain on the scalp for too long. This may sound like a difficult process, but each time you apply a relaxer to your daughter's hair it will become easier and easier.

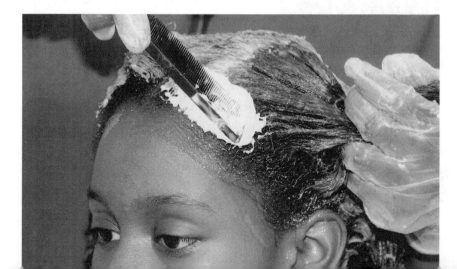

RELAX:
Timing Is
Everything

● ● ● ● ●

The entire application process should take about twenty minutes, depending on the length and thickness of the hair. Watch your time and try to work fast enough to completely cover and mold the entire head.

Always save the hairline area for last; it is the most sensitive and the easiest to irritate. Make sure you apply a sufficient and even amount of relaxer to your daughter's hair.

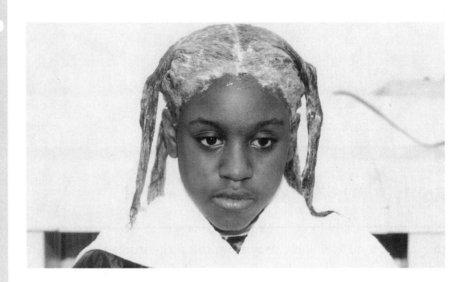

Molding the Hair

Take the very first section that you applied relaxer to, and with the back of the comb or with your gloved fingers, rub the relaxer deeper into your daughter's hair. Repeat this process throughout her entire head, section by section, in the same order in which you applied the

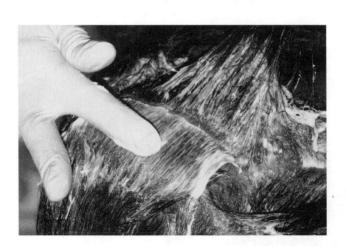

relaxer. If you see any hair that does not have relaxer on it, put some there, especially around the hairline. Make sure you ask your daughter how she's feeling again. If she says that her scalp is itching, that means that within the next two to five minutes the relaxer may start to irritate her scalp and it will be time to rinse out her hair, even if you are not quite ready to do so.

Rinsing, Shampooing, and More Rinsing

Now it's time to rinse, which is a very important step. Give your daughter a towel to cover her eyes. Start to rinse her hair where you applied the relaxer first, unless there is an area that your daughter says is hurting or burning, then rinse this area first with cool water, using low water pressure. Make the water temperature warmer and quickly proceed to rinse the remainder of the relaxer out of her hair.

Use warm water and gently move your hands through your daughter's hair to help break up the relaxer and control the flow of the water. You don't have to finish one section before you move to the next, but you do want to move briskly through the hair. Rinse, rinse, rinse, and rinse some more until the water runs totally clear.

Once the water runs clear, begin to shampoo your daughter's hair with the neutralizing shampoo. You should shampoo at least three times just to be sure all the chemical has been removed. Then rinse well and apply the conditioner. Leave the conditioner in for ten to fifteen minutes, and then use a wide-tooth comb to comb through the hair.

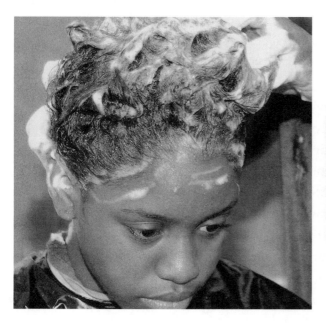
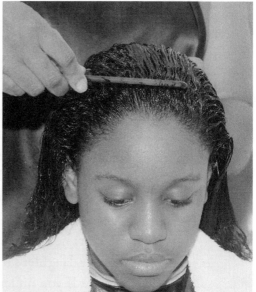

Just a reminder: if you rinsed and shampooed your daughter's hair in a forward direction over a sink, continue to comb her hair in this direction until you have done your final rinse. Gently towel-dry your daughter's hair and apply a leave-in conditioner. You can also apply a setting lotion or wrapping foam to help you style her hair.

I recommend that your daughter's ends be clipped after her first relaxer, then as needed. It makes the hair healthier and more manageable and helps it stay in place longer.

Remember, if you didn't get your daughter's hair as straight as you wanted, you'll have plenty of other chances to try again.

Styling Your Daughter's Hair

Now you and your daughter have more styling options. You can go beyond braids, and on special occasions, you can use rollers or curling irons to create bangs. You can either dry her hair with a hood dryer or a blow-dryer, or you can still let her hair air-dry in braids or pigtails.

Blow-drying is not a method that should be used too frequently because too much heat can damage the hair. If you do use a blow-dryer, put it on a medium heat setting, and before you begin, allow the hair to air-dry a little or remove most of the moisture from your daughter's hair with a towel.

If your daughter's hair is very long or thick, it is best to dry it in sections. Use a blow-dryer that has a comb attachment and dry one section at a time. It will be easier to work from the bottom to the top of her head; the hair dries more quickly this way. After you have dried your daughter's hair, you may apply her favorite hairdressing cream.

If you prefer to use a hood dryer to style your daughter's hair, you can braid the hair or roll it up in plastic or mesh rollers. With either method, first apply setting lotion, then place your daughter under the dryer until her hair is completely dry. After your daughter's hair has dried, you may spray her hair and scalp with an oil sheen

RELAX:
Time for a
Touch-up

When your daughter's hair becomes hard to comb from the root area, it's time for a touch-up.

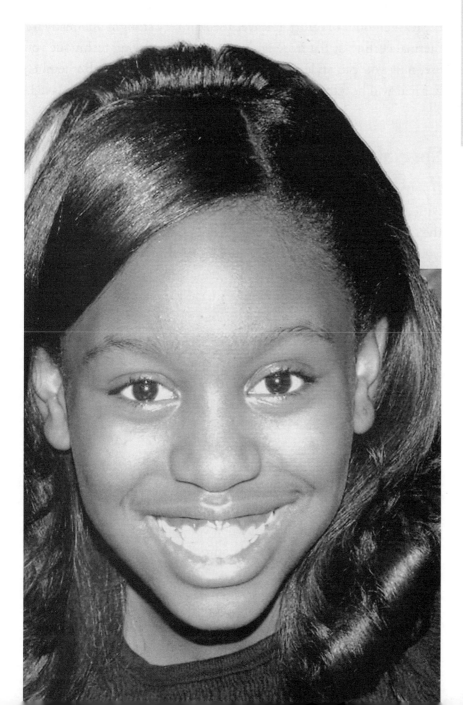

spray or apply a little oil. Then gently massage the oil into her scalp to stimulate hair growth.

Or, depending on your daughter's age, you may want to try the wrapping technique. Wrapping is often recommended for preteen girls because of the various styling options that can be achieved. With the least amount of effort, it leaves the hair very straight and ready for thermal curling or flat ironing. No matter what drying technique you use, now you can style your daughter's hair as she likes. Remember, her hair will be a little more fragile after it's been chemically relaxed.

Special Care for Relaxed Hair

If you want to protect the beautiful hairstyle you've created, tie it up with a satin scarf or a hairnet at night; another option for protecting the hair is to use a satin pillowcase. Older girls will probably be more conscientious about keeping their hair well maintained. Under no circumstances should you let your daughter go to sleep with hair ornaments in her hair. They can damage her hair as she twists and turns during the night.

Now that your daughter has relaxed hair, in six to ten weeks she will need to get what is called a touch-up. That means the new hair that grows out from her scalp will need to have relaxer applied to it. The timing for your daughter's touch-up will depend on the texture of her hair and how fast it grows. Typically, hair grows about half an inch a month.

The steps for doing a relaxer touch-up are similar to those for applying the first relaxer, except now you will be applying the relaxer primarily to the new growth. Also, if portions of her hair did not get as straight as you wanted them when you did the first relaxer, this is a good time to comb more relaxer onto those areas. Be careful—you don't want to overprocess the hair.

If you have overprocessed your daughter's hair, take her to a professional hairstylist right away. If you can't get to a hairstylist,

RELAX:
Over-processing

● ● ● ● ●

You can tell when your daughter's hair is over-processed because when it's wet, it feels like wet cotton, and when it's dry, it breaks like dry spaghetti.

purchase a protein reconstructive treatment, which you will need to apply for at least two months or until the hair begins to feel stronger. The breakage will decrease as the hair becomes stronger.

Relaxer Application in Thirteen Steps

1. Apply the protector cream (base) along the hairline, continuing around the perimeter of the head and behind the ears. Be sure to cover the earlobes and the neckline as well.

2. Part the hair into four jumbo sections and apply the protector cream onto the scalp using quarter-inch partings, then secure the sections with hair clips.

3. Mix the relaxer according to the manufacturer's instructions, using the wooden spatula that's included in the kit or something plastic (never use metal). Let the mixture sit.

4. Start the application process on the back left or back right crown section.

5. Take a quarter-inch to a half-inch section of hair and apply the relaxer one inch away from the scalp, stopping about half an inch from the ends. Try not to get any relaxer on the scalp.

6. Flip the hair over and apply the relaxer to the back side of the hair. Work neatly and swiftly.

7. Take another small section and continue to apply the relaxer in the same manner.

TIPS FOR RELAXERS

- ▶ Relaxers are not recommended for girls under eight years old.

- ▶ Always try to use kiddie relaxers on girls between the ages of eight and twelve for straighter hair.

- ▶ Always read the manufacturer's directions.

- ▶ Never put relaxer on an unhealthy scalp (one with sores, bruises, or cuts).

- ▶ If the relaxer starts to burn, rinse the area immediately with cool to lukewarm water using low water pressure, then rinse the rest of the head with warmer water.

- ▶ Always rinse and shampoo the hair thoroughly.

- ▶ Always condition the hair after shampooing.

- ▶ Caucasian straighteners and African American relaxers are two totally different chemicals and are not interchangeable.

- ▶ When in doubt, seek professional help.

8. Be sure each section is thoroughly saturated with the relaxer before moving on.

9. Follow steps 5 through 8 for the other crown section and the two front sections.

10. Save the hairline and nape areas for last; they are more sensitive than the rest of the hair.

11. Start molding the hair in the area where you first applied the relaxer. Using your fingers or the back of the comb, smooth and rub the relaxer into the hair in quarter-inch sections.

12. After rinsing the hair thoroughly, shampoo it two or three times to get out all the relaxer.

13. After shampooing and conditioning, the ends of the hair should be clipped. Then you will be ready to style it.

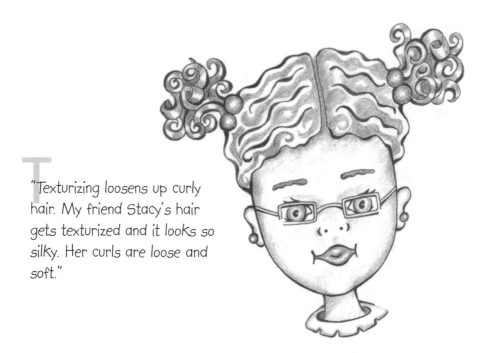

"Texturizing loosens up curly hair. My friend Stacy's hair gets texturized and it looks so silky. Her curls are loose and soft."

Texturizing Curly Hair

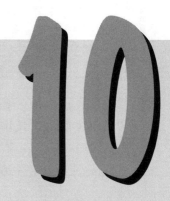

10

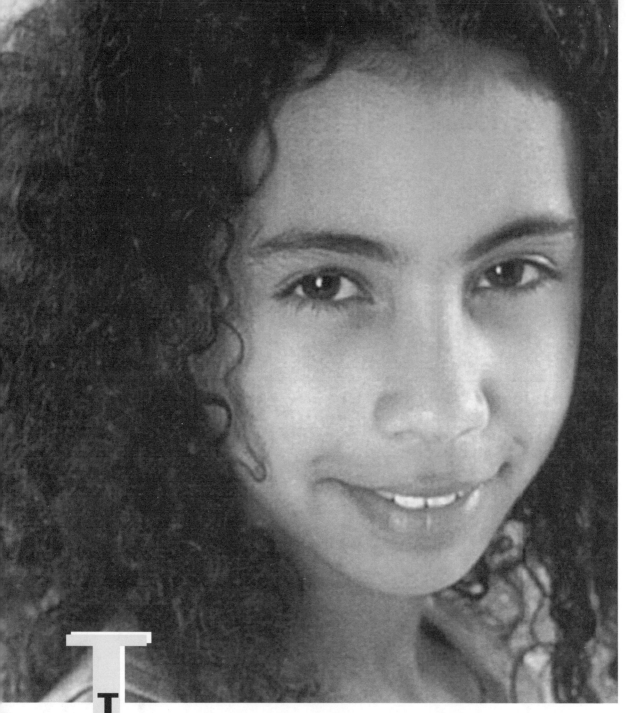

Texturizing can make a world of difference, especially on hair that is thick and curly. It will help tame the hair so that it is easier for you and your daughter to comb through it and control the curl. It will not remove all of the curl from the hair, but it will loosen up the curl and remove some of the thickness and frizz.

First you need to know what kind of relaxer or texturizer to purchase. The type of relaxer that you are going to use is a little different from one used for kinky or excessively curly hair, but it is still a safe relaxer.

This particular relaxer contains sodium hydroxide lye, which means that you will not have to mix anything together in order for

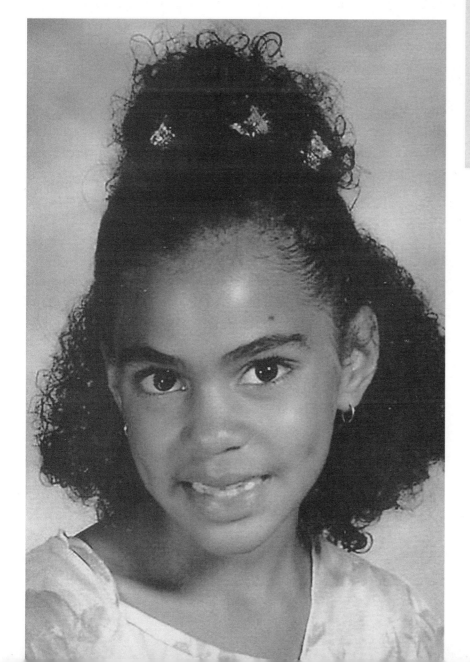

DON'T TAKE ANY CHANCES

● ● ● ● ●

Wait until your daughter is at least ten years old before you texturize her hair. If your daughter's hair is so thick and unruly that you need help, find a professional hairstylist.

it to work. Although you can later use a kiddie relaxer kit, if this is the first time you are texturizing hair, it's better to use a sodium hydroxide relaxer. I have listed some relaxers of this type in the back of the book.

If you put a sodium hydroxide relaxer into your child's hair, she cannot have a straightener meant for Caucasian hair, like Thermal STR8, put into her hair. This would cause serious breakage.

In most cases, lye relaxers are not available in kits. You will need to buy a neutralizing shampoo and a conditioner, but try to use products that are all of the same brand. You will also need a pair of plastic or rubber gloves, a wide-tooth comb with a handle, and some hair clips to hold the hair. Make sure you have your towels, shampoo, and conditioner all in place. You should also have chosen your method of rinsing the hair and have all related items ready. Finally, read the manufacturer's instructions thoroughly.

Step 1: Examine Your Daughter's Scalp

First, examine your daughter's scalp for any sores, abrasions, or other openings. Ask her if she has been scratching her scalp; if she says no, then you're good to go. If she has been scratching, wait twenty-four to forty-eight hours before proceeding.

Step 2: Get Prepared

Apply the scalp protector around your daughter's hairline, on the top of her ears, and to the back of her neck. Drape a towel around her shoulders.

Step 3: Mix and Apply the Product

Open the relaxer and stir it with a wooden or plastic object (a spatula, a knife, or a spoon) to balance out the chemicals in the jar. Part the hair into four jumbo sections: straight down the middle, then across the top, from ear to ear. Secure each section with a hair clip. Start the application process in the area where you feel the hair is most unruly.

Take your comb and dip it into the relaxer, then comb the relaxer onto the section of hair you have selected first. Next, gently comb the relaxer onto that section, staying about half an inch away from the scalp. Repeat this step on the next section of hair, which should be directly underneath the section that you just finished. Work in a neat, orderly pattern; don't jump from one spot to the next. Keep the sections of hair small to make your job easier.

The whole texturizing process involves simply combing the relaxer through the hair. After you have completed the entire head, let the relaxer sit. The amount of time the relaxer stays on the hair depends on how long it takes you to apply it and how thick or curly the hair is. To loosen up the natural curl in very thick and curly hair usually takes from thirty to thirty-five minutes, including application time. When your daughter's hair looks like it is straight, it's time to rinse out the relaxer.

Step 4: Rinse, Shampoo, and Condition

After rinsing thoroughly, shampoo the hair at least three times using a neutralizing shampoo. Then apply a deep, penetrating conditioner to the hair and let it sit for ten to twenty minutes. Finally, rinse out the deep conditioner and apply a leave-in conditioner.

Step 5: The Final Comb-Out

Comb the leave-in conditioner through your daughter's hair, then remove the moisture from her hair with a towel. Apply antifrizz or curl-control products, comb the hair, and let it air-dry. If you can't let the hair air-dry, use a blow-dryer with an attachment called a diffuser. This dries the hair without blowing it around and will keep the curls in place.

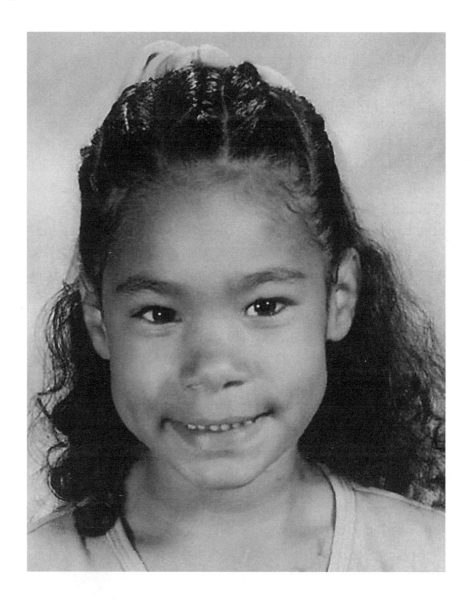

As with relaxing, it's a good idea to trim your daughter's ends after her hair has been texturized. Because her hair is straighter, cutting it should be easier.

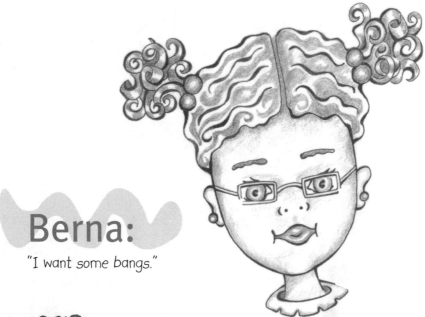

Berna:
"I want some bangs."

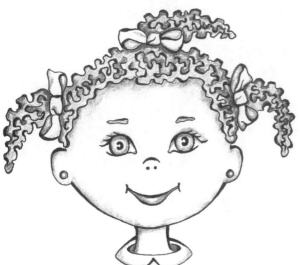

Lula:
"Then you will have to sleep with a roller in your hair, if you want them to stay curled."

Curls: Tools and Tips for Your Daughter's Hair

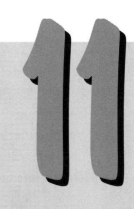

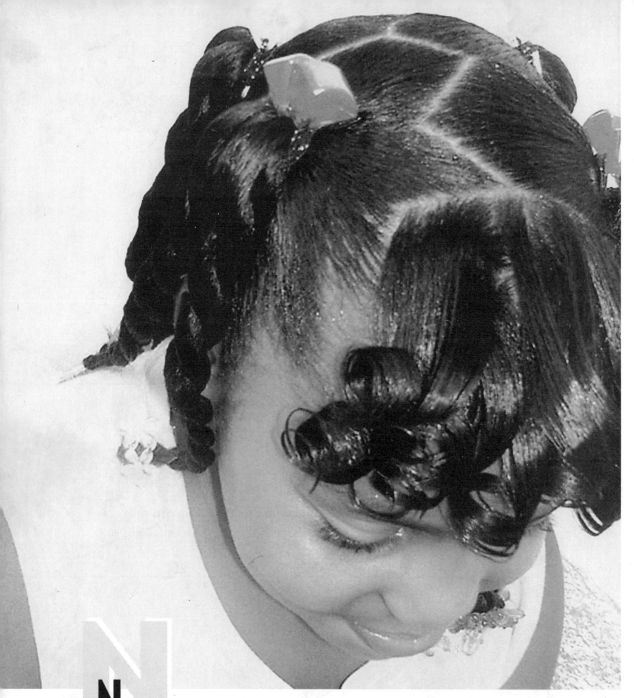

Now that your daughter is older, she may be begging for curls in her hair. Conventional thermal irons, like the ones that our grandmothers and great-grandmothers used, are made of steel and have a heavy, round, solid-steel bar. They are heated by being placed on your gas or electric stove or in a ceramic stove, like the one used by professional hairstylists.

Since we are talking about your young child's hair, I see no reason why you should use a thermal curler, unless it is a special occasion and you want your little girl to wear a headful of curls. Even if your daughter is a preteen who likes to wear her hair down, it will be better to use other curling devices, such as rollers, until she gets older.

Using hot irons too frequently will cause the ends of the hair to become dry and brittle, resulting in split ends. Pressed hair can probably withstand heat from the curling iron better than relaxed hair. So handle relaxed hair with extra care and avoid using excessive amounts of heat on it.

Curling Irons and Flat Irons

When using curling irons or flat irons on the hair, use hair maintenance products designed for heat. Many hair companies make

DON'T TAKE ANY CHANCES

● ● ● ● ●

Flat irons and curling irons can damage a young child's hair. Don't curl or flat iron your daughter's hair too often. Save it for special occasions.

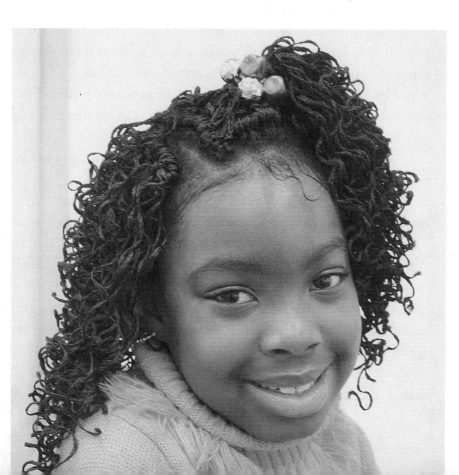

DON'T TAKE ANY
CHANCES

● ● ● ● ● ● ●

When used incorrectly, curling irons and flat irons can burn the hair and the skin. Test the iron on white tissue paper before using it on the hair. If the tissue paper turns brown, the iron is too hot and can damage the hair.

products just for this purpose; they seal the cuticle and act as a protective shield for the hair. Many types of curling tools can be used to create some really nice hairstyles for your daughter.

Conventional curling irons or marcels are small, so they produce smaller, tighter curls. Unless you have used these irons before, you may not want to take on the challenge. Using them requires some skill. They can also do extreme damage if they are used on chemically processed hair.

Thermal curling irons are used most frequently. They are also made of steel and come in a variety of sizes, from micro to jumbo. The barrels on most of these irons are hollow so that they will not be heavy, and they heat up more evenly. Just like the conventional marcels, these irons must be heated using external heat from a stove. Always test thermal curling irons before using them. If you know how to use a thermal curling iron properly, you can create beautiful silky curls. Different thermal irons can create spirals or crimps or further straighten the hair.

Flat irons can help preteens have smooth, silky hair. They come in a variety of sizes and should be used in moderation and very carefully.

Crimping irons produce pretty waves on the hair. They can be made of steel and come in several different sizes.

Electric curling irons have a spring handle, and some have a marcel grip. Irons with the marcel handle or the long handle are the ones that most African American stylists use. You can use electric or thermal irons on hair that has been blow-dried, pressed, or chemically straightened.

Many nonprofessionals use curling irons with the spring grip because they are easier to maneuver. Electric curling irons are available in a variety of sizes, from small to jumbo, and some have a temperature control setting. When using electric curling irons, you should check to see how hot they are before applying them to the hair. The medium setting is pretty safe to start off with on most textures of hair.

Ceramic curling irons are the newest and latest thing in hot styling tools. Curling irons that are made of ceramic are said to be better for the hair. They hold the heat more evenly and put less stress on the hair. There are also ceramic flat irons, or straightening irons, which are used to smooth and produce silky-straight hair.

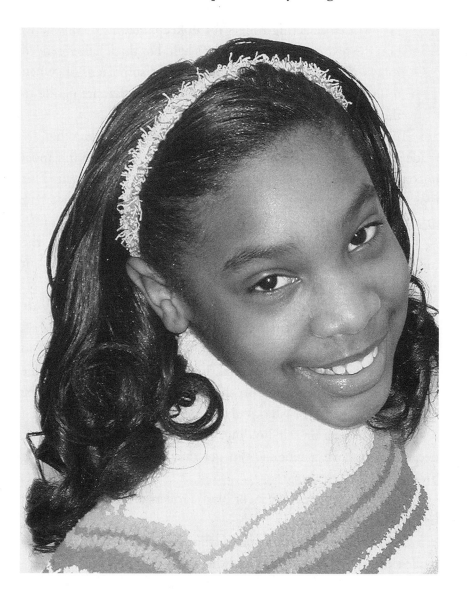

DO YOUR
RESEARCH

● ● ● ● ●

Rollers come in a variety of sizes, materials, and shapes. Some require bobby pins or hair clips to secure them, and some have two parts: the roller and the fastener.

Hair Rollers

Hair rollers can be used in a couple of different ways. Some can be used for wet sets, and some can be used for upkeep. Hot rollers come as a set and should be used on dry hair. Hot rollers must remain in the hair for about thirty minutes in order to create curls. There are also hot rollers that are microwavable.

When selecting rollers for upkeep, take into consideration the texture of your daughter's hair. For thick hair you need rollers that fasten securely and provide some tension when rolling. For thin hair you should use rollers that are gentle to the hair.

To keep things simple and safe you should use rollers that are made of nonabsorbent material. Plastic hard rollers are the most uncomfortable to sleep in, but they are the safest for the hair. This type of roller also works best when you sit your daughter under a hair dryer.

Foam rollers are great for sleeping in, but they absorb the moisture from the hair. Use these rollers with end papers to prevent absorption.

Satin foam rollers should work well for your daughter. They are easy to sleep in and the satin covering helps protect the hair.

Wire-mesh rollers are also safe for the hair but are difficult to sleep in. They must be secured with hair clips or bobby pins. Some wire-mesh rollers have small brushes inside them. These should be removed because the brushes pull out too much hair.

Velcro rollers or self-holding rollers are not the best option, because they have a tendency to get tangled in the hair, causing breakage.

Snap-on magnetic rollers or plastic rollers are safer for the hair but are hard to sleep in.

Pillow rollers are soft rollers that are designed for comfort while sleeping. They wrap around the hair.

Soft-twist rollers are long, skinny tubes and come in several different sizes. I would not recommend sleeping in these rollers, but they do make pretty spiral curls.

There are also spiral rods, perm rods, and crimping rollers, all of which are very hard. None of these is recommended for sleeping, but they can be used for setting the hair in tight curls.

So what should you do to your girl's hair at night? You can roll her hair with satin foam rollers or pillow rollers, wrap her hair, or do pin curls. (Steps for wrapping hair and doing pin curls follow.) Then tie a satin scarf or a bonnet around your daughter's hair. Be sure to select a scarf or a bonnet that fits your child's head correctly; you don't want one that is too big (it will slide off as she sleeps) or too tight (it will hurt). You will find satin bonnets, wraps, and hairnets wherever African American hair products are sold.

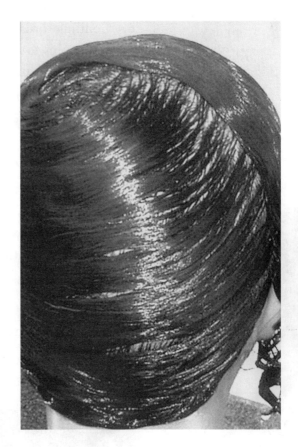

Hair Wrapping in Seven Simple Steps

1. With a wide-tooth comb, comb the hair straight down and part it on the left or right side of the head.

2. On wet hair, use a comb to comb a section of hair toward the part. On dry hair, use a brush to do the same thing.

3. Comb or brush another section of hair around and into the previous section.

4. Continue this same method, traveling around the head.

5. Comb or brush the hair from the other side in the same direction, wrapping the hair around the head.

RELAX:
Oiling the Scalp

● ● ● ● ● ●

I believe in applying oil or moisturizer to children's scalps whenever necessary, especially if the child has dry hair or a dry scalp.

6. Continue brushing or combing the hair around. You can use bobby pins to hold the hair in place, especially if you are doing this on dry hair.

7. Tie a satin scarf or a bonnet around your daughter's head to keep the hair in place.

Pin Curls in Five Fast Steps

1. Take a small to medium section of hair.

2. Placing your index finger on the scalp at the base of the section of hair you're working with, loosely roll the hair around your index finger until you come to the end of the strand.

3. Slide the hair off of the finger. It should lie flat on the scalp.

4. Secure the hair with a bobby pin.

5. To secure the hair for the night, cover it with a satin scarf or a bonnet.

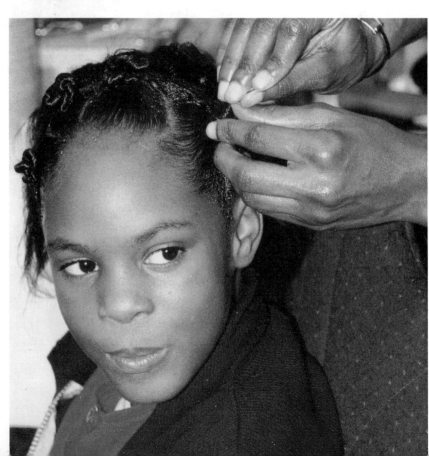

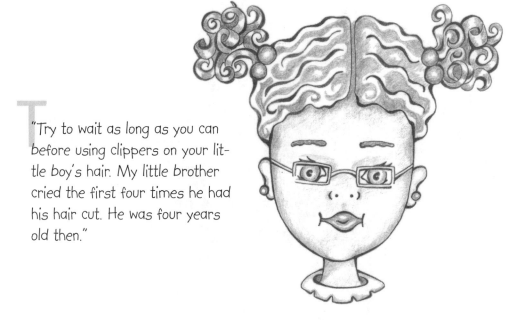

"Try to wait as long as you can before using clippers on your little boy's hair. My little brother cried the first four times he had his hair cut. He was four years old then."

Hair Care for Beautiful Little Boys

12

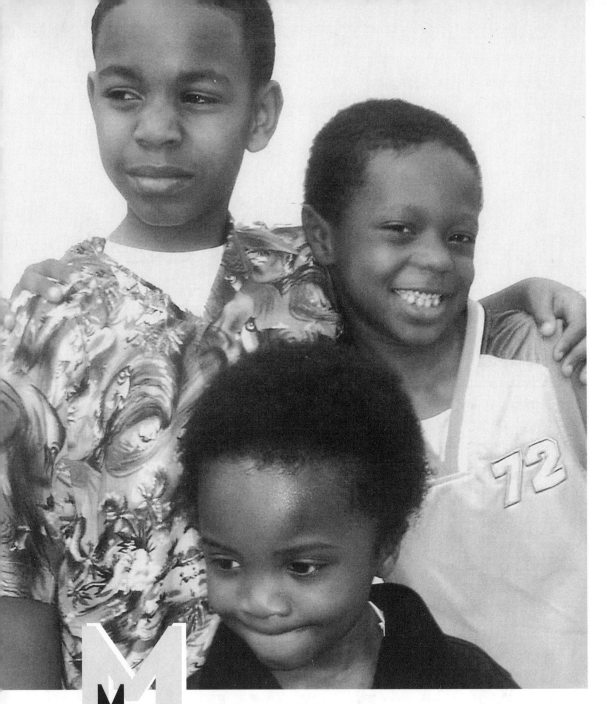

Most of my friends tell me that they are so glad they had a son, because if they had a daughter, she would have to live with me. When it comes to hair, little boys can be a breeze, even when they do not like getting their hair combed. With boys the most important task is keeping their hair clean, brushed, combed, oiled, and neat as much as possible.

One topic that I have not yet talked about is the occurrence of a very thin or bald spot in the back of the head. This is a common problem among African American infants—boys in particular. It's caused by the friction that happens while your baby is lying on his back. Usually, as the child grows and is able to sleep in different positions, his hair begins to fill in.

Infant to Two Years Old

If you have a baby boy, until he is two years old you should treat his hair just as you would treat your little girl's hair. Wash your son's hair with the same mild baby shampoo, and if it is hard to comb, run the same cream rinse or conditioner through it.

DON'T TAKE ANY CHANCES

If your baby develops a bald spot from lying on his back, massage the back of his head as often as possible to increase circulation and encourage new hair growth.

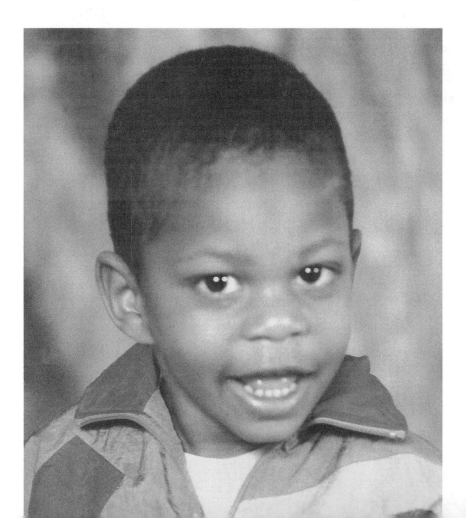

Always shampoo and towel-dry your son's hair with a white face-cloth or hand towel. Next, apply a small amount of oil to his hair and scalp; then brush or comb his hair in the direction that it grows.

Hair texture plays a key role when deciding what you can or cannot do to your son's hair. Some parents like to braid their little boy's hair and let it grow long; that is entirely up to you.

Two to Four Years Old

For little boys with a tight curl to a kinky curl pattern, follow the same shampoo and conditioner procedure that you would with a little girl that age. Be sure to comb his hair out thoroughly with a wide-tooth comb before it dries.

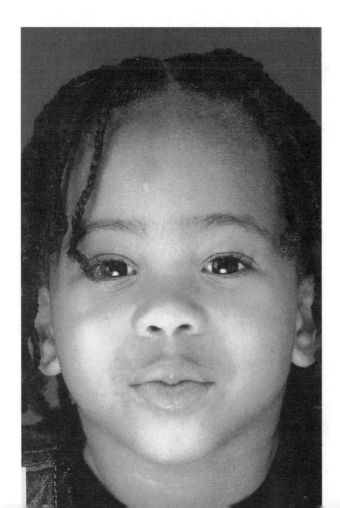

To trim or cut your son's hair, use a hair pick and then use medium-size, sharp scissors. When your son reaches the age of three, you may choose to have his hair cut with clippers, or you can just continue to cut his hair with the scissors. Read the chapter on cutting your child's hair for more information. Of the two cutting methods, clippers are more difficult to use. You should probably take your son to the barbershop for his first haircut.

After your son's hair has been clipper cut, shampoo it and then oil his scalp. This is especially important if his hair has been cut down to the scalp. Always make sure you keep your clippers clean.

Some parents may choose other style options for their sons with very curly or kinky hair, such as braids or locks. If you choose locking for your boy's hair, you can do it by taking a small section of the hair and twisting it or palm rolling it. This has to be done on a daily basis until the hair grows longer and the locking process becomes easier. Just like other natural hairstyles, locks and braids must be shampooed and conditioned at least biweekly.

If your son's hair is wavy or curly, at this young age you should still use a mild shampoo. There are no rules that say how you should or should not style his hair. If your son's hair has gotten too long for you, I recommend cutting it wet, right after you have combed it out.

The key to a successful cut is to cut a small amount first, and then comb it, cut, then comb, and cut again. This way you can see exactly what your son's hairstyle looks like.

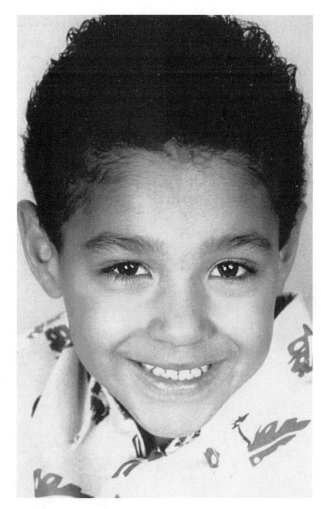

Remember, wavy and curly hair shrinks when it starts to dry, so to keep it even, make sure it stays a little damp while you are cutting. If you prefer, you can cut the hair dry and then shampoo it. After cutting, add a little oil or hair moisturizer as needed.

Four to Twelve Years Old

By the time your son reaches the age of four, you will have basically trained his hair. Keeping his hair clean and conditioned is the most important thing you can do for him. The styling will come easy as he grows. Either continue using the same techniques and styles that you used when he was three, or experiment with different variations of combing, trimming, cutting, braiding, or locking; but please, no chemicals.

Have fun with your beautiful little boy's hair and he will grow into a handsome, well-groomed teenager.

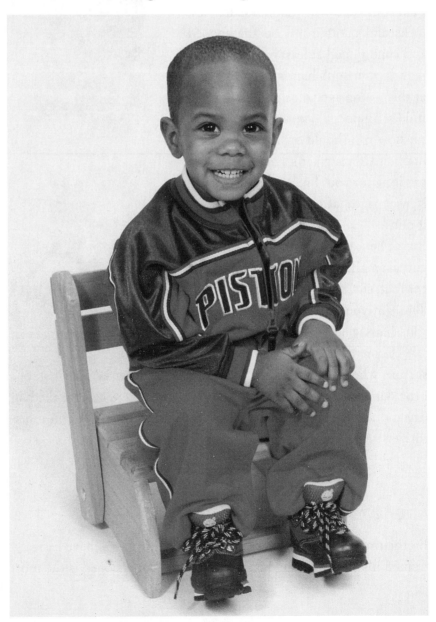

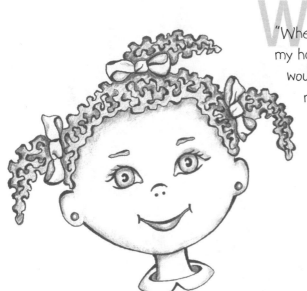

"When I get older I want to wear my hair down. Mom said my ends would have to be clipped and made even."

The Pros and Cons of Cutting Your Child's Hair

13

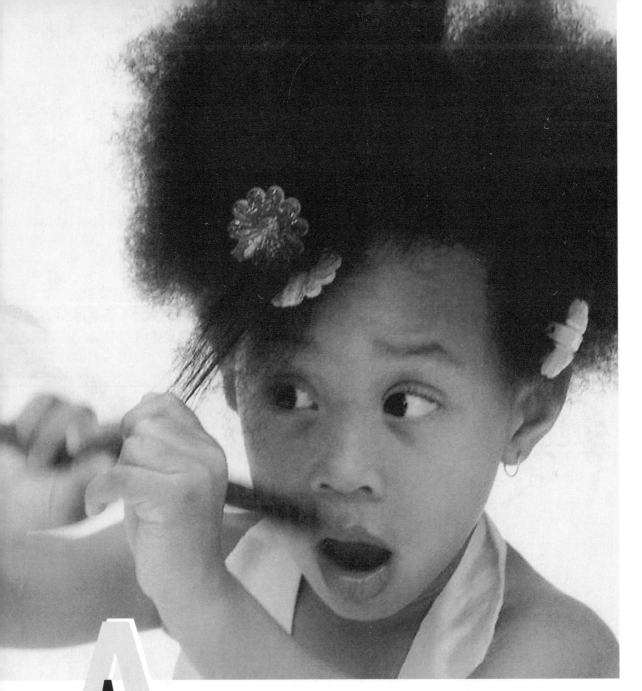

All parents need to know how soon their child's hair should be cut. Some parents assume that cutting their young child's hair will make it grow faster and healthier. Perhaps, but again, it all depends on the texture of your child's hair and the purpose for cutting it. You may want to cut it to achieve a particular style or to remove damaged ends.

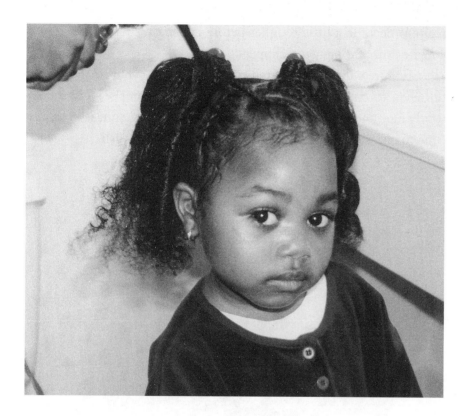

Although I recommend waiting until your child is at least three years old, age has very little to do with when you should cut your child's hair. Cutting the hair can make it more manageable, cause less tangling, and make the ends of the hair healthier.

In the case of our girls, it all depends on the child's hair texture and your own personal likes or dislikes. If the ends of your daughter's hair are extremely dry and uneven, or if she has received a chemical relaxer, her hair needs to be trimmed.

Most of us decide that we want to cut our boys' hair because it makes it easier to manage, but the decision to cut your son's hair is a personal choice. What will help you decide is the way you want your son's hair to look and the texture of his hair.

If your infant son has very kinky or wool-like hair, you should try to wait until he is at least two years old, closer to three, if possible. Young scalps are very tender, and it's better to wait for your son's scalp to become a little tougher before cutting his hair, especially if you are going to be using clippers.

Texture will be key when it comes to making your final decision on when to cut your son's hair. For instance, if your son has kinky, wooly hair and braiding is not an option for you, then it is probably time to cut his hair when it's too long to comb or brush.

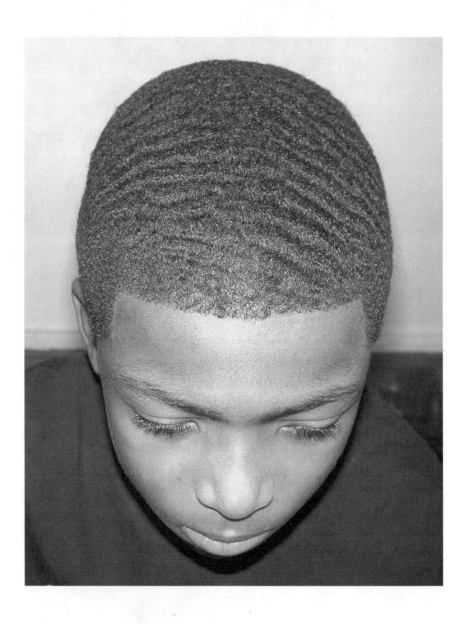

If your son has curly or wavy hair, then you may want to lightly trim his hair. You can take on the challenge by trimming or cutting it yourself or take your son to a salon or barbershop for that first haircut.

For those of you who would like to do it yourself, I provide step-by-step instructions starting on page 111. You will need scissors, combs, a pick, clippers with guards, and a haircutting cape or a towel.

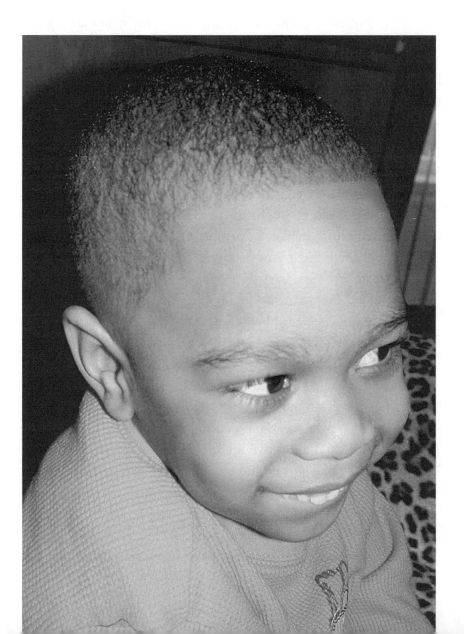

DO YOUR RESEARCH

So, when should you cut your son's hair? It's all up to you and your son, but here are a few facts that may help you with your decision:

- Does he look like a girl instead of a boy because his hair is so long? If you want him to wear it long, cut it close on the sides or in the back (nape area) to give him a more boyish look.

- Is it time for him to start school? Some schools have dress codes.

- Is his hair matted or badly tangled? Maybe you can't comb out the tangles and you have to cut them out.

- Is his scalp unhealthy or hard to keep clean and fresh? Boys should shampoo their hair more often then girls because they have a tendency to get really dirty and they sometimes sweat in their hair.

If you plan to cut your son's hair for the next couple of years, you should invest in a pair of haircutting shears. You can purchase a decent pair of shears at a beauty-supply store or a discount chain store for $9.95 to $19.95. You don't need to spend a lot of money on them. To keep them in good condition, don't use them to cut anything other than hair.

Haircutting shears come in different blade lengths. For cutting little ones' hair, four to six inches are a good length. For cutting older children's hair and for cutting afros, five- to seven-inch shears will work. You should also choose your shears depending on hair texture, hair thickness, and your level of comfort while using them.

When you purchase your combs, touch the tips of the teeth to make sure they are not sharp. The combs that you select should be made from hard plastic or hard rubber. For cutting hair, use a wide-tooth comb for removing tangles from the hair as well as a haircutting comb. A haircutting comb has both narrow and wide teeth; it is used for cutting, removing smaller tangles, and smoothing the hair.

Picks can be found where African American hair products are sold and are good for both kinky and curly hair. For children, I prefer to use plastic picks. Choose one that fits your hands and can handle the amount of hair that your child has. The thicker the hair, the larger the pick should be.

If you want to try cutting your son's hair close to the scalp and up to two inches long, clippers will do the job more quickly and more easily than scissors. They can be purchased as a packaged set, which includes the clippers, guards, oil, combs, and scissors. Clipper guards are used to help achieve the length you want. The larger the teeth of the guard, the less hair you will remove. The smaller the teeth, the closer you will get to the scalp and the more hair you will remove. Some clippers have adjustable blades. The level on the side of the clippers moves the blades up and down; the lower the blade, the shorter the hair will be.

Using clippers takes a little practice, so start with the large guard first. If you want a faded look or a very tapered, clean look, I strongly recommend taking your son to the barbershop.

You also need a clip to help hold your son's hair out of the way when you are using scissors, particularly if he has three or more inches of hair.

Lastly, get a haircutting cape to cover up your son while you are cutting his hair. You can also use a towel or a small sheet, if you have to. When hair has been cut, it has a tendency to stick to clothes and skin; this can be very itchy. Just in case, use a small clean towel with some talc or baby powder on it to help remove the cut hair from your son's skin and clothes.

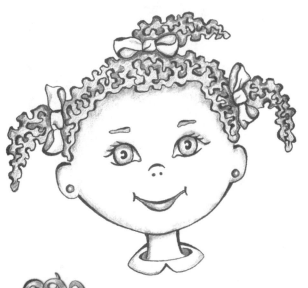

Lula:

"A girl in my class cut her own hair."

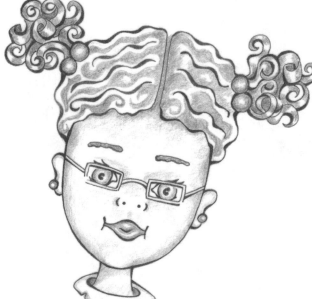

Berna:

"What happened?"

Lula:

"She had to go to the beauty shop so they could fix it. It's cute, but it's shorter. She said she won't do that again."

Let's Cut Some Hair!

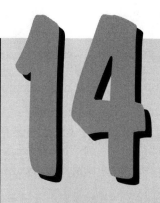

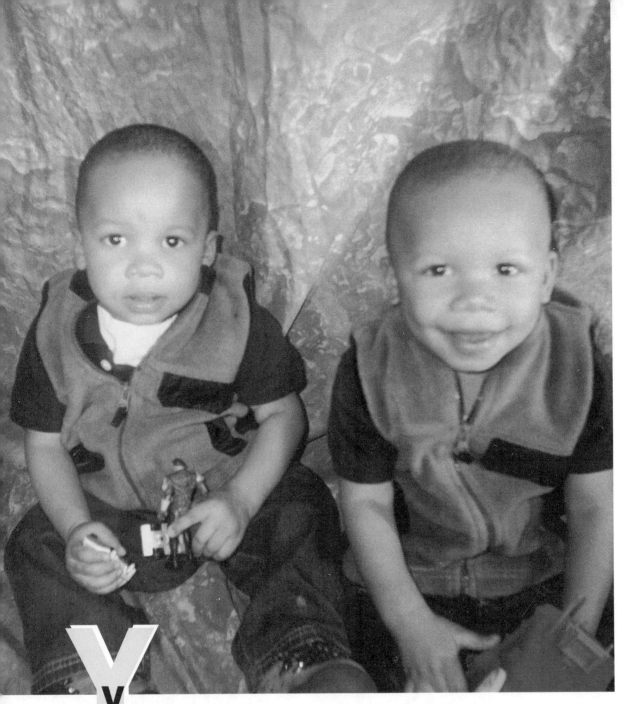

Your little boy is two and a half to three years old, and it's time for a haircut. Sit him in a chair that will put his head at the height of your stomach or chest. Make sure the back of the chair is not higher than his head. It works best if the back of the chair reaches up to the top of your child's shoulders, so you may want to sit him on a couple of phone books.

Talk to your son; tell him what you are about to do. Don't be alarmed if he tells you in a really loud voice: "No! No! I don't want a haircut!" That's when you'll have to get creative, reminding him about Daddy, an uncle, a brother, or any male who gets haircuts whom he knows and likes. Once you have prepared your son emotionally and mentally, give him something to look at or play with. Make sure it will keep his head up and his eyes focused forward.

If Your Son Has Kinky Hair

For kinky hair, use either a pick and the freehand cutting method (using scissors) or clippers. On young scalps, I prefer scissors, especially if this is the first haircut. The freehand method is the easiest to learn and the most mistake proof. Unless your son has been going to the barbershop while Daddy gets his hair cut, clippers will probably frighten him.

Step 1. Cover your son with a cape or a towel. Use a clip to secure it around his neck. You can put a towel underneath the cape also. It prevents the hair from sticking to the neck.

Step 2. Pick the hair out as much as you can. If the hair has not been combed in several days, you should use a wide-tooth comb to remove the tangles first. Do not apply oil to the hair or the scalp prior to cutting; it causes the hair to stick together and makes it harder to cut. Use the pick to comb the hair from the scalp to the ends. Pick, pick, and pick some more until you have the hair standing straight up all over the head like a big, bushy afro.

Step 3. Starting at the top of your son's head, begin to cut the ends, working from the crown to the front. You will probably have to hold his head in order to keep him still. Gently hold your son by his chin and talk to him while you are cutting his hair; you can stand in front of him while doing this.

Work your way over to the side after you have cut the hair on the top and when it looks somewhat even. Work your way over to

LESS STRESS

Before you begin to cut your son's hair, ask yourself if he will be able to sit still long enough. If not, you may want to wait until he's a little older or take him to a professional.

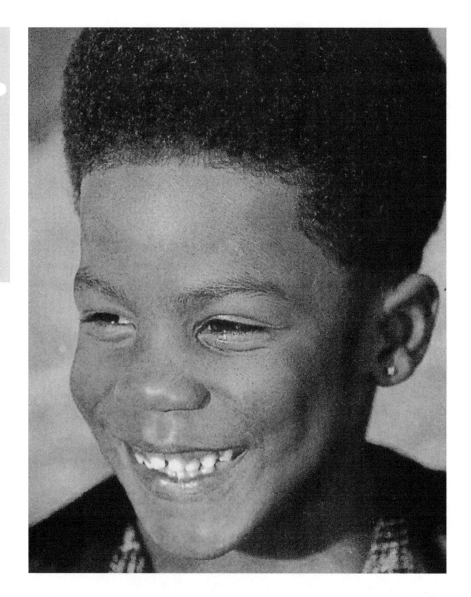

DON'T TAKE ANY CHANCES

● ● ● ● ●

Clippers can cause cuts just like scissors. To be safe, it might be a good idea to skip shaping the hairline until your son gets a little older.

the opposite side and then to the back. Your first run will be to make the hair look a little even. Now you're going to pick the hair out again and repeat the whole process. Do this until the hair looks even all over and when you are satisfied with the length of the hair.

Step 4. The hairline area is usually shorter and can give the hair a nice polished look. Cut around the hairline very carefully, making sure you don't snip his ears.

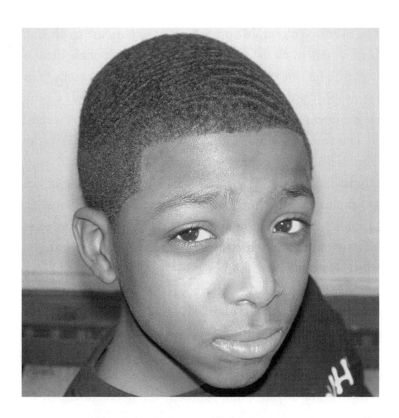

If Your Child Has Curly or Wavy Hair

You will need the following tools: scissors, combs, spray bottle, cape, shampoo, and conditioner.

Curly hair comes in many different varieties. A child can have soft, loose curls, medium-size curls, tight curls that are soft, or big curls. No one has the same texture of curls, and a variety of textures can exist on one head. Depending on the tightness of the curl, the thickness of the hair, and your level of confidence, you can either pick the hair out and cut it as if it's an afro, or you can wet the hair down and do a scissor cut. Since we have already talked about cutting hair when it's dry, let's look at how to do a wet cut on a boy or a girl.

Step 1. It's a good idea to shampoo your child's hair first or, if the hair is already clean, wet it using a spray bottle. To make combing easier, pour some detangler into the spray bottle along with the water; half and half is a good combination.

Step 2. Cover up your child and get out your haircutting shears; five-inch blades will work as well as four-and-a-half-inch blades. Comb your child's hair in the direction that it grows. Normally, hair on the top grows forward and the rest of the hair grows down. Comb the hair straight down all the way around the head, like a mushroom.

Step 3. The first cut will be at the front, from the crown to the forehead. You can use the nose, the eyes, or the eyebrows as your guide. Comb the hair on the top of your child's head, directing it forward, toward the forehead. Hold a one-inch section of hair between your index finger and middle finger. Glide down to where you want to make your first cut. You will see the bad ends; this is what you want to remove. Your hands should be positioned over the forehead, nose, or lips, depending on the length of the hair. Now cut just beneath your fingers. Hold your child's hair with some tension but not a lot as curly hair bounces back.

Step 4. Return to where you started; comb a small section of hair that you just cut along with a new hair section of hair. Let the previously cut hair act as your guide, and cut the new hair the same length. Continue this method all around the hairline, always checking where you are in reference to the head. If you are by the ear, you can cut this hair a little shorter because it leads into the back of the head. This hair can also be cut longer if that is your preference.

Once you reach the back of the head, return to the front and cut the other side, going in the opposite direction from where you started. This helps you achieve a more even cut. If it's not totally even, don't worry; you can fix it later. Remember, this is curly hair, and the curls are going to do their own thing anyway. Your goal is to just get rid of some of the length and make the hair look neater.

Step 5. Now you want to cut the rest of the hair. Starting at the top of the head, from the crown, pick up a one- or two-inch vertical section. Cut the first section of hair as much as you think is needed. Moving toward the forehead, pick up another section of hair, along with some of the hair you just cut. Cut the hair in the same way you cut the previous section, taking the section between your middle and index fingers and cutting just above your fingers.

Step 6. Go back to the crown area where you started. You're going to circle around the head, using the crown as your center point, until you have cut the hair all around your child's head.

Step 7. You are just about finished. Now comb the hair the way you want your child to wear

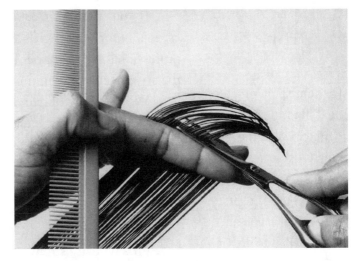

it. Because the hair is curly, it is not going to look perfect, but if you see an area that is still too long, just take a small vertical section, pull it down toward the shorter hair, and cut it equal to the length of the shorter hair; this will blend the top hair, or longer hair, with the shorter hair.

When you have finished the cut, put some moisturizer or light oil on your child's hair.

Is It Necessary to Trim Your Daughter's Hair?

You may wonder why you sometimes see different lengths of hair on your daughter's head. Some of her hair may be in the growth stage, some may be in the resting phase, and some may be in the replenishing, or shedding, phase. Also, certain areas of the hair grow faster than others.

Eventually all hair needs a good trim or a cut, but it depends on your daughter's hair and your long-term goals for her hair. There is one rule of thumb to follow: always make sure you cut the ends of your daughter's hair after a relaxer.

LESS STRESS

● ● ● ● ● ●

For some pointers, the next time you get a haircut, watch the hairstylist to see how he or she holds the hair and the scissors. This will give you an idea of what to do. Or check out a haircutting tape.

If you want your daughter's hair to have a particular style, especially for young girls with wavy or curly hair, take her to a professional stylist for her first styled haircut. Then you can keep the style neat by trimming it every six to eight weeks.

What texture of hair does your daughter have? For instance, with wavy and curly hair, split ends have more of an adverse effect on the rest of the hair. Unhealthy ends travel up the hair strand, so it is best to cut them off. This will help make the hair look better, feel better, and hold a style, and will prevent continued splitting of the ends.

Kinky hair reacts differently to uneven ends, especially on little girls who are still wearing their hair in braids. Notice that I said uneven ends; there's a difference between uneven ends and split ends. The ends will be uneven because hair grows at different rates. If the ends become split, tangled, or dry, they need to come off. This will allow the rest of the hair to stay healthy.

For young girls, up until around the age of ten, if you see that their ends are unhealthy, you can trim them. This works best on curly-kinky to kinky hair. Simply braid your daughter's hair into ten or twelve braids, depending on the thickness of her hair, and snip about a quarter to a half inch off each braid. This will remove the worst of the ends without removing too much length.

Purchase the Correct Tools

If trimming your child's hair is something you plan to do for the next couple of years, purchase the correct tools:

- Wide-tooth comb
- All-purpose or haircutting comb
- Shampoo
- Conditioner
- Towels

- Cutting cape
- Hair clips or butterfly clips
- Spray bottle for water
- Scissors (haircutting shears)

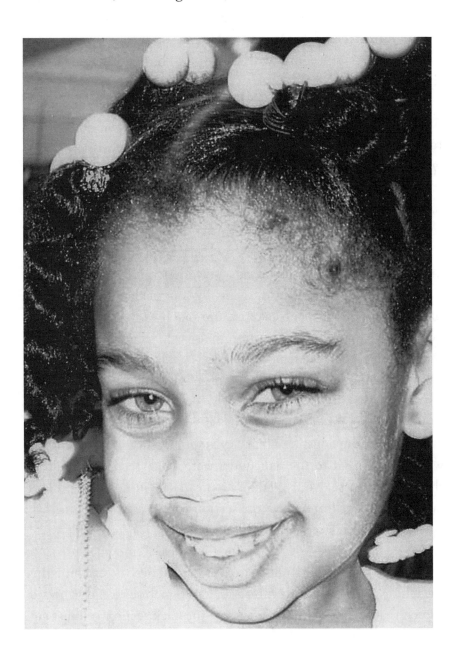

DON'T TAKE ANY CHANCES

● ● ● ● ●

How does hair get split ends? If you comb the hair with the wrong tools, apply heat too frequently to the ends of the hair, don't cover the hair at night, or just don't take care of the hair.

Trimming Your Child's Hair

This method of cutting is for straight, wavy, or curly hair that comes below the earlobes or longer. It is a basic haircut that will clip the ends of the hair only. If the hair is shorter, you may use the technique previously mentioned for cutting curly hair (see page 111).

Control is the most important factor when cutting hair; following these procedures will allow you to have more control over the hair.

Step 1. Shampoo and condition the hair. Depending on the texture of your child's hair, it can be cut wet or dry. If the hair is fine textured, cut the hair dry. If the hair is thick, cut it wet. If the hair is worn pressed, then press the hair first.

Step 2. Section the hair into four parts, straight down the middle and across the top, ear to ear. Use butterfly clips to secure each section into a small knot.

Step 3. Starting in the back two sections, comb down about a one-inch section of hair from each side, directing it straight down. Caution: hair in the nape area is usually shorter than the rest of the hair, so you don't want to take off too much of this hair. You may need to take down another section to use as your guide. This hair is usually longer than the nape hair, or the "kitchen hair" as we used to call it. Starting in the center, trim off about half an inch or more, whatever you think is needed; it is always best to remove less first.

Step 4. Comb another section of your child's hair downward, and using the previously cut hair as your guide, cut the section of hair while matching it to the hair underneath. Your sections should be thin enough to see your guide underneath. Continue this process, taking more hair from above the section you have just cut until you have cut both back sections.

Step 5. You are now ready for the sides. Remember to try to keep your child's head straight up. Starting above the ear on either the left or the right side, comb about a one-inch section downward. Match that section with the length of the back section you just cut.

Comb the hair straight downward, match it up to the previous section, and cut it. If the sides are shorter than the back, you will need to cut the sides on an angle. Take another thin section, using the previously cut hair as your guide. Continue until you have cut the entire side. Then start on the opposite side. If the hair on top of your child's head does not reach all the way down, you will have to do a little bit of vertical cutting.

To vertically cut, comb the side hair downward. From the center part down to the ear, make a one-inch vertical section. Hold the section vertically, slightly elevating the hair. You will see the ends that need to be trimmed and you should match them to the previously cut hair.

Step 6. To make the style look even better after you have cut both sides, take one-inch sections in the crown area, hold the hair straight up, and cut off the ends as needed.

Congratulations! You have completed your child's trim; now you can style the hair.

If you are not comfortable with trimming your child's hair at home, take him or her to a professional. Make sure you tell the stylist that you would only like to have your child's ends trimmed, not a haircut. Please remember, hair grows according to heredity and how well it is taken care of. Healthy ends are always a good thing. Good luck!

"I don't like peas, carrots, green beans, spinach, greens, or brussels sprouts. Yuck! I do like lettuce, but I do not like most vegetables, so my dad gives me a fruit shake that tastes really good. He says it is good for me because it is very nutritious."

Feed the Body, Nourish the Hair

15

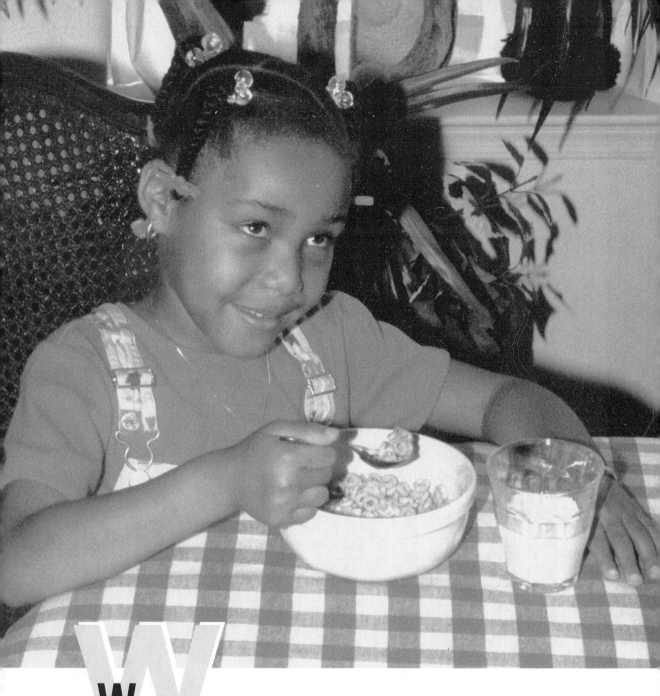

We all know that a healthy diet is important for our children. But getting children to eat what we want them to, in many cases, can be a problem. We either have children who like to eat everything or those who are very picky. An unhealthy diet can contribute to hair breakage, slow hair growth, dry hair, and hair loss. The best way to feed the hair is to feed the body properly.

A good way to give your child a healthy body is to balance the essential nutrients, such as fats, carbohydrates, proteins, minerals, and vitamins. If you do this and still feel your child is not receiving proper nourishment through his or her diet, you may want to give your child a multivitamin. Some doctors don't prescribe multivitamins for children, so check with your child's pediatrician to see what he or she recommends. No matter what you and the

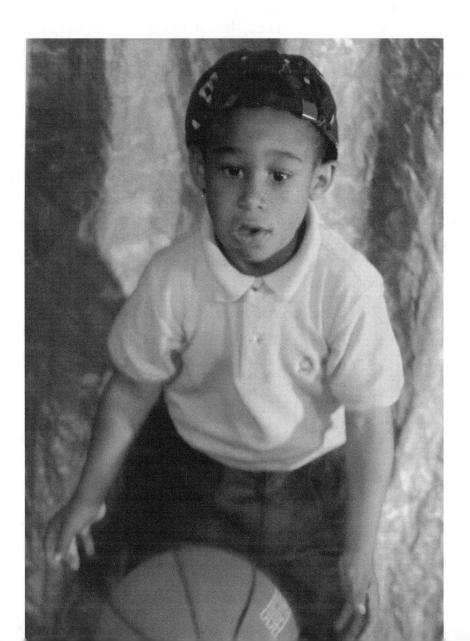

pediatrician decide about vitamins, it is essential to feed your child good, balanced meals that contain many of the vital nutrients he or she needs to stay healthy.

Starting your child's day with a healthy breakfast is always very important, so try to prepare a meal that your child will enjoy, like a nice bowl of oatmeal with raisins, which are rich in iron. You may want to alternate the oatmeal a few days a week with an egg and cheese sandwich on whole-wheat bread; add some ketchup or whatever condiment your child likes. Many studies have shown that children who eat breakfast perform better in school and have more energy than children who do not eat breakfast.

Since hair is made of protein, foods rich in protein will contribute to healthy hair and skin. You should regularly serve your child protein-rich foods, such as poultry, oatmeal, lean red meats, and seafood, as well as foods that contain iron, zinc, copper, and iodine. Make sure your child is receiving all the vitamins a growing body needs. Foods that are rich in B vitamins include cheese, eggs, fish, whole grains, beans, peas, and leafy green vegetables. Vitamin A is found in sweet potatoes, broccoli, cantaloupe, and papaya.

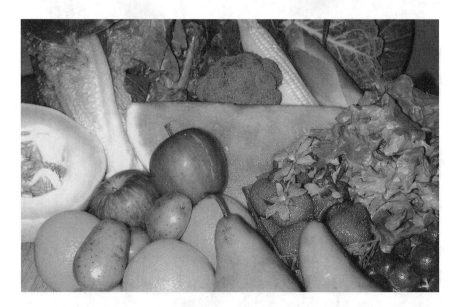

Foods that have vitamin C are very important as well, and include citrus fruits, tomatoes, melons, and strawberries. Calcium-rich foods like cheese, milk, kidney beans, and yogurt are also recommended for your child's diet.

Whenever possible, we should avoid giving our children foods that are high in fat or sugar, and we should minimize their intake of starches and fried foods. Children who are sluggish have slower blood circulation, which doesn't promote healthy bodies and hair. So by starting your child off on a healthy diet, you are forming a foundation for continued healthy eating, which is beneficial in many important ways. Occasional treats, like ice cream or a Happy Meal, are fine. Always remember, a nutritious diet puts your child on the road to becoming a healthy, happy, and productive human being.

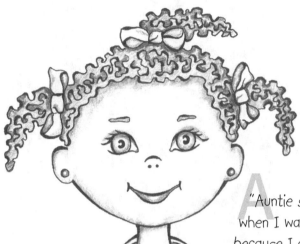

"Auntie showed me a picture of me when I was a baby. It didn't look like me because I didn't have any hair. I was bald. She said I had something called 'cradle cap,' and it took my hair out. I asked her why did I sleep in my cradle with a cap on? She laughed and said that's not what it means. She said my mom took me to my doctor and she gave her some medicine for it, and then my hair started to grow back. Boy! Am I glad I have some hair now."

Understanding Your Child's Hair Loss

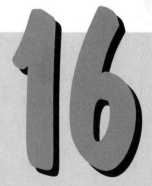

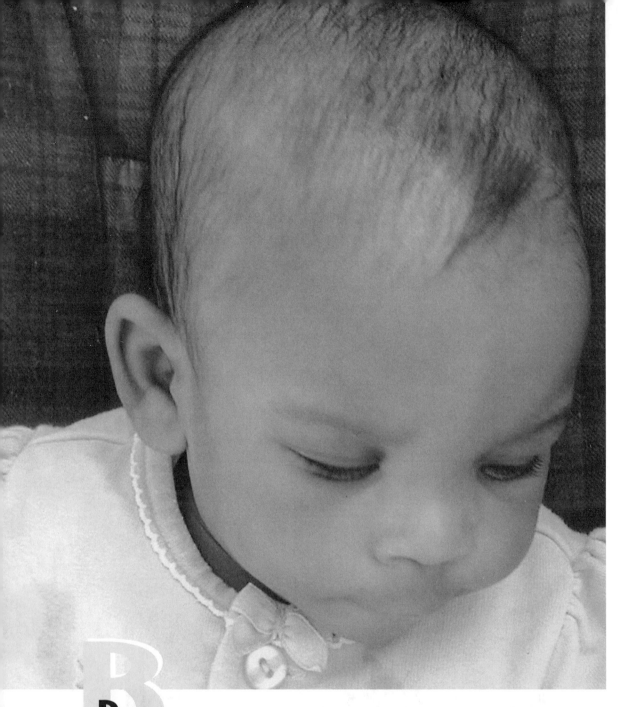

Breakage of your child's hair or bald spots on his or her scalp can occur for many reasons. Although breakage is rare in the case of infants, if it is occurring, it is more than likely due to health reasons. Here are a few possibilities to consider:

If you are breast-feeding, your child may not be receiving the proper nutrients from your breast milk because your diet is deficient in something. Perhaps you are lacking iron in your system. What goes into your body also goes into your child's body.

The problem could be the hat that you are putting on your child's head every day. Make sure your child's hats are clean, and stay away from materials that may irritate the scalp, like scratchy wool.

Is your child on any medication? Some medications can cause hair loss; consult your pediatrician.

Maybe the fault is in the air; a very dry environment can cause dryness in the hair.

Do you apply too much oil to your child's hair and scalp? Too much oil clogs up those little pores.

Do you shampoo your child's hair with an adult shampoo or soap? That's not good, either. Adult shampoo is often too harsh and drying to a young child's hair and scalp.

Are you using a baby comb that has sharp teeth? Be aware that sharp teeth can tear babies' fine hair and hurt their tender scalps.

Does your child share a comb and brush with someone else? Bacteria, oil, and dandruff are only a few reasons why you should not share combs and brushes.

Is someone else combing your child's hair, perhaps a day-care provider or a relative? Find out what they are using and how they are doing it. That could be a contributing factor to your child's problem.

Hair Loss in Newborns

Many newborns are born with a head full of hair, but within one or two months, that hair falls out and is replaced with new hair. This is natural. However, if you continue to see hair loss and no new growth, consult your child's pediatrician.

Don't worry if your child has a bald spot on the back of his or her head. Hair in this area often grows slower because children rest and sleep on their backs. The hair eventually grows back in as your child grows older.

Cradle Cap (Infantile Dermatitis)

Cradle cap appears as scaly or patchy yellow flakes that are sometimes greasy. It does not itch or cause the baby distress. Doctors say that this condition of the scalp is harmless and not due to infection, allergy, or poor hygiene; the cause is unknown. Some doctors believe that the mother's hormones stimulate the sebaceous glands on an unborn baby's scalp, causing cradle cap to develop.

Eventually cradle cap goes away, but it can become severe and spread to the baby's face, eyelids, or trunk. If this happens, seek medical help. Doctors usually treat severe cradle cap with very mild hydrocortisone cream and a special shampoo.

If your child develops cradle cap, I recommend loosening it by rubbing the area very gently with a comb or a brush. After loosening the cradle cap, shampoo your child's hair twice with a mild baby shampoo.

After rinsing and towel-drying the hair with a white towel, take a cotton swab or ball, rolling it in your hand first to remove loose cotton fibers, and use it to apply a small amount of witch hazel to the area. (You may saturate the cotton with water if you feel the witch hazel may be too harsh for your infant's skin.)

Finally, apply a small amount of castor oil to the area. This aids in healing. Severe cradle cap can cause long-term problems, so if the condition persists, take your child to a dermatologist or a pediatrician.

Managing Hair Loss in Children Ages Two and Above

In older boys and girls, aged two to ten, there are many reasons for breakage or bald spots. I have listed some below:

- Harsh or too-strong chemicals
- Dry scalp and hair

- Emotional or physical stress
- Tight ponytails and braids
- Illness
- Medications
- Wool and straw hats
- Chlorine
- Excessive dryness or oily dandruff
- Improper diet
- Not shampooing the hair often enough
- Leaving the hair uncombed for too many days
- Using too many or excessively harsh products, like heavy, waxy grease and heavy hair gels
- Using unclean combs and brushes
- Not combing the hair thoroughly from the roots to the ends
- Leaving extensions in the hair too long
- Eczema or ringworm

Handling Hair Loss with Your Sick Child

In most cases, if your child becomes ill and loses his or her hair, it will grow back. During treatments like chemotherapy, hair loss often occurs. The hair does grow back, but hair loss can be difficult to cope with, especially for girls. If your daughter has hair loss for an extended period of time, wearing a wig might help her feel better about her appearance. If so, there is a nonprofit organization that will help you through this trying time. Locks of Love provides hair-pieces to financially disadvantaged children under age eighteen who are suffering from long-term medical hair loss. For further information, visit their Web site at www.locksoflove.org.

Conclusion

My mission in writing *Wavy, Curly, Kinky* was to make the daily hair care routine more enjoyable for you and your child. I also wanted to explain variations of our hair textures and methods of styling your African American child's hair.

I hope this book has helped you in some way; perhaps it has shown you a new technique or answered a few questions. By no means are my ways the only ways, but they are time-tested, healthy ways toward helping your child grow the most beautiful head of hair possible.

If you have any questions or comments, please e-mail me at drl.art@sbcglobal.net.

Appendix A
What If?

I call this section "What If?" because some of you may have these questions, and I have heard them all and experienced all of the answers.

Q *What if I realize that I need some hair cream and don't have any around the house?*

A Try your favorite body lotion or moisturizer; it always works in a pinch.

Q *What if my child's hair is drier in the winter than in the summer?*

A Depending on where you live, winter weather can wreak havoc on anyone's hair. If you live in an area that gets cold and snowy, then your child is probably going to have dry hair. Cold and dry air takes away much-needed moisture. Also, your child likely wears a hat on winter days. Most winter hats are made from wool, acrylic, or a blend, all of which also take moisture out of the hair. Try finding a hat that is lined with silk or satin to protect the hair. Using a moisturizing conditioner or a hot-oil treatment will also help.

Q *What if my child's hair is matted?*

A The hair becomes matted if it has not been combed on a daily basis or if proper drying techniques are not used after it is shampooed. Sometimes, your little girl's hair gets matted from the playground or your son comes home with his hair in a mess from a rough football game. Hair that has been unbraided will mat if not thoroughly combed out, especially if the braids were small or cornrows. If you find yourself facing a clump of hair, apply a small amount of conditioner, detangler, or cream rinse directly to the tangled area. Let the product sit for a few minutes and then slowly and gently loosen the knot, using the first tooth in a wide-tooth comb or the tail of a rattail comb. Be sure to hold the hair at the root area, and then start to remove the knot, strand by strand.

It is going to take some time, so be patient and give your child something to play with or read. If it's in the morning and you are in a hurry, try to style the hair around it. Maybe you can put your child's hair in a ponytail or a puff and leave it until you have the time to remove the knot properly. If you have tried and tried to remove the knot and you can't get it out, then your only recourse is to take a small pair of scissors and snip a few hairs at a time, combing as you go. Eventually the knot will loosen.

Q *What if my child likes to go swimming a lot?*

A Swimming is fun, and in the summertime when it's hot, there's nothing as cool as going swimming. I remember going to the neighborhood pool at least three times a week. I would wear a swimming cap, but my pressed hair would get a little wet or, more often, a lot wet. It would depend on how long I stayed in the water, or if some knuckleheaded boy pulled my cap off. My hair would end up smelling like chlorine.

As an African American child who loved to swim, there was no way I could shampoo my hair every day. I would just rinse it and braid it. Today there are shampoos designed to remove the chlorine from swimmers' hair. Even with these shampoos, most swimmers' hair will become dry and sometimes brittle, depending on how often they swim.

If you apply conditioner or hair grease to the hair prior to swimming, it cuts down on the amount of chlorine that is absorbed into the hair. Of course, it is always a good idea for your child to wear a swim cap. Regardless, the hair should be rinsed each time your child swims and shampooed at least once a week. Always give the hair a deep penetrating moisturizing conditioner and a hot-oil treatment when you have the time.

Q *What if I have shampooed my child's hair and I discover that I don't have any conditioner or detangler?*

A As a quick fix, you can spray some liquid fabric softener onto the hair, then add a small amount of body lotion. This will soften the hair and leave it smelling really fresh.

Q *What if my child puts a pound of hair oil, grease, or Vaseline into his or her hair?*

A I cannot tell you how many times I have heard this story. The first thing you should do is wipe out as much of the oil as you can with a paper towel. Then go out and buy a cleansing or clarifying shampoo. Next, use talcum powder, baby powder, or baking soda and apply it throughout the hair, massaging it well into the hair and scalp. Finally, rinse the hair well in warm water and shampoo with the cleansing or clarifying shampoo. These shampoos have more cleansing power and should always be followed with a conditioner and leave-in treatment.

Q *What if my child's hair has gum in it?*

A Apply ice to the gum and then remove it. If you are going to shampoo the hair right away, you can use peanut butter to remove the gum and then it will slide right off.

Q *What if my child always sweats in his or her hair, especially during the summer months?*

A Children play hard in the summer, and their little bodies release heat in the form of sweat through their heads, but a little sweat isn't so bad. For little boys, when you bathe them or have them take a shower, give them a light shampoo. If there is dirt, grass, or bugs in their hair, as there often is, two latherings will probably be needed. After a thorough rinsing, apply a little moisturizing conditioner, towel-dry the hair, and apply hair oil.

Boys' hair is pretty easy to deal with, but for little girls who sweat in their hair, it depends on the texture of the hair. Some girls' hair is wash and wear, and some hair needs more care, especially if it is pressed or relaxed. If you don't have time to shampoo your daughter's hair right away, you can temporarily cleanse the scalp by rubbing witch hazel or Sea Breeze on it.

If you want to cleanse the hair more thoroughly, you can use a no-rinse shampoo or cornmeal. Yes, I said cornmeal! Cornmeal was used many years ago by African Americans in the South, where they did not have access to shampoo and water. You simply apply the cornmeal in one-inch sections to the scalp and then, using a boar-bristle brush, brush the hair from the roots to the ends. Continue this process until you have gone through the entire head and until no more cornmeal is present. This works as a temporary method to freshen up stale hair.

If the hair really needs to be thoroughly cleansed, of course you should always shampoo and condition it as soon as possible.

Q *What if I don't like my child's hair color, or my child wants to change his or her natural hair color for some reason?*

A Coloring your child's hair can cause a lot of damage to his or her hair and scalp. And what if your child has an allergic reaction to the color?

But, let's just pretend it's Halloween and your child is dressing up in some kind of costume and really wants to look the part. Here are a few ideas and products that you can safely use to temporarily color the hair.

Temporary hair-color spray is found in cans and comes in a variety of colors. Before you apply the spray, coat your child's hair with a small amount of oil to cut down on the amount of color that is absorbed into the hair. Sometimes these colors are hard to shampoo out, so don't use too much spray.

As a precaution, always cover any exposed skin and your child's clothes with something disposable, like paper towels. Make sure you apply the spray in a well-ventilated area, and always read the manufacturer's directions before you use it. Remember that anything from an aerosol can is flammable.

Baking soda or cornstarch works well on little African American boys who want to make their hair white. It does create a little dust, but it's safe.

Crepe hair is found in most costume shops and comes braided in a variety of colors. To use it, remove the braid from the package, take one strip of hair at a time from the braid, and begin to pull the hair into little strands. As you work with the hair, it starts to become frizzier and fuzzier looking. The more you work the hair, the more it starts to look like kinky hair. Continue this process, adding more hair as you go; eventually you will have enough to put on top of your child's hair.

You will need to secure the crepe hair, so either use a hat, if it's part of the costume, or tie some string around your child's head and then cover the string with the hair, or you can use hair pins.

You can use eye shadow to give your little one a color effect in his or her hair. Try a streak of blue, white, purple, or red; it washes right out.

A cheap wig is probably the quickest and easiest solution to changing your child's hair color instantly.

Highlights are okay if your child is in the entertainment industry and you want to add a little color for effect. If you do, take him or her to a good hairstylist who knows about coloring African American hair. Please don't let anyone color your child's entire head of hair; a few strands here and there are all that you should allow to be done.

Q *If my daughter wears braids all the time, does she need to have ends cut?*

A If your daughter's hair is being maintained properly, the result will be healthy hair and growth. Braided hair doesn't need to be cut unless the ends are really bad. On the other hand, split ends, matted hair, and tangled ends will cause the hair to become more damaged if they are not removed. If your daughter has received a chemical service or you are trying to achieve a particular hairstyle, such as bangs or a bob, some cutting will be required.

Q *What if the hairstylist wants to trim my daughter's hair every time she gives her a relaxer or a retouch?*

A If your daughter has received her first relaxer, have the ends trimmed then. Relaxed hair must be taken care of in a different way. The structure of the hair has changed, and it is not as strong as natural hair. So it is very important to remove the ends after a relaxer has been applied.

Q *What if my daughter is in a wedding, a beauty pageant, or a talent contest, but her hair is short. What styling options do I have?*

A This is a really fun and exciting time, and you have gone all out to make sure your daughter looks very special. Her hair will be an extremely important part of her whole appearance, so here are a few styling options.

You can take your daughter to a professional hairstylist and explain how you want her hair to look. You can have your daughter's hair braided with extensions. Depending on your daughter's hair texture, you can go to a beauty-supply store and buy some hairpieces in different styles. Take your daughter to the store with you and pick a hairpiece closest to her hair color and texture. It's not necessary to buy a very expensive piece of hair. Bring the hairpiece home and then cut it down to fit your daughter's head. Secure it with hairpins.

A great way to style your daughter's hair is to pull all her hair back and make a ponytail. Or what about bangs? Add a pretty hair ornament around her face and wow! She'll look like a little princess.

Appendix B
Some Products to Try

You can usually tell a good product by its feel, its smell, and sometimes its price. If it just sits on top of your hands, then it will probably just sit on top of the hair and the scalp. When you rub the product, it should melt slightly into your skin. Avoid products that contain a lot of wax and fillers. It is best to try different products because they react differently on different textures of hair and in different climates. Here are some of my recommendations:

Very Light Oils
TCB Lite Hair & Scalp Conditioner
New Era Feather Touch Light Hair and Scalp Treatment

Light to Medium Oils
Beautiful Beginnings Oil Moisturizer (contains vitamin E, aloe, and natural oil)
Baby Love Moisturizing Creme Hairdress
PCJ Pretty-N-Silky Creme Oil Moisturizer (contains Vitamin E)
Just For Me! Scalp Conditioner and Hairdress

Oils for Dry Hair
Fantasia IC Deep Penetrating Cream Moisturizer
Baby Love Moisturizing Hairdress Lotion
Just For Me! Creme Conditioner & Hairdress
Beautiful Beginnings Scalp Conditioner & Hairdress
Kemi-Oyl
Lustrasilk Moisture Max
African Royal Castor G.R.O.

African Royal Mink Oil Gel
Optimum Care Nourishing Creme Hairdress

Products for Hair Pressing
LeKair Cream Press
Dudley's Curling & Pressing Wax
Ultra Sheen Creme Satin Press
Lustrasilk Hair Culture Solution

Kiddie Shampoos
Baby Love line of products
Gerber Baby Moose Foaming Wash
Johnson & Johnson Baby Shampoo Moisturizing Formula

Mild Shampoos for Children 8 to 12 Years Old
Crème of Nature Herba Rich Soft Cleanse Shampoo
Sheenique Silk Moisturizing Shampoo
Always Natural Shampoo Moisturizing Formula
African Royale BRX Braid Shampoo (a super-softening
    herbal shampoo)

Kiddie Relaxers No-Lye Kits
PCJ
Beautiful Beginnings
Just For Me!
Motions for Kids

Relaxer Maintenance Products
Motions for Kids line
PCJ line
Beautiful Beginnings line
Just For Me! line

Sodium Hydroxide Relaxers
Optimum

Designer Touch
Revlon Realistic

Cream Rinses and Detanglers
Feels-Like-New Detangling Rinse
Just For Me! Leave-in Conditioner
PCJ Daily Pretty-N-Silky Detangling Spray
Paul Mitchell The Detangler
Infusium 23, Original Formula Pro-Vitamin Leave-in
    Hair Treatment
Infusium 23, Moisturizing Formula Pro-Vitamin Leave-in
    Hair Treatment
Crème of Nature Regular Formula for normal hair
Crème of Nature Ultra Moisturizing Formula for dry,
    brittle, or color-treated hair

Dandruff Products
Neutrogena T/Gel line
Glover's Medicated line
Paul Mitchell Tea Tree special line
Sulfur 8 Medicated line

Products for Braids and Natural Hair
African Pride
Dark & Lovely Naturally
Organic Root Stimulator

Hair Ornaments
Scünci
Girl Gear

These are not the only products that you can use, but you should always look for products that are of good quality.

APPENDIX C
Recommended Tools

These are some of the tools that I have used that are of good quality and safe for the hair.

Scünci combs and brushes
Diane combs and brushes
Boar-bristle brushes
Wahl clippers
Andis clippers
Conair Styler Dryer 1875, model number SD4BLR

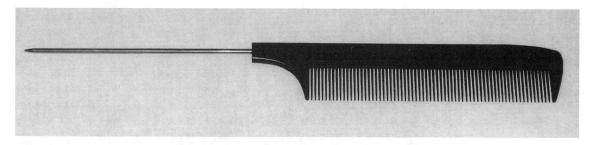

This rattail comb with metal tip is very good for undoing braids, especially skinny ones.

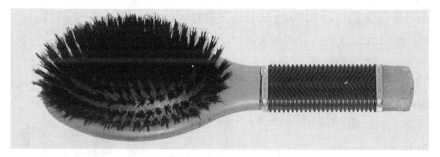

A boar-bristle paddle brush is good for smoothing out the hair.

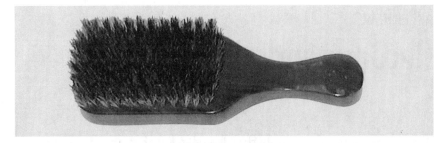

A flat boar-bristle brush works well on boys for smoothing out their hair and making waves.

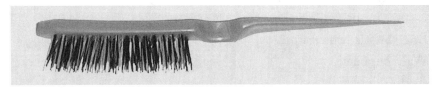

This small plastic brush is one of my favorites; it has many uses. For young girls, it works well on fine hair and really helps smooth out the edges along the hairline.

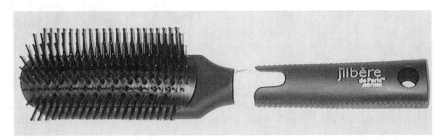

This brush has hard plastic teeth and can be used when blow-drying the hair or on wet hair to remove tangles. It works well on many different textures of hair.

This plastic brush can be used on medium- to fine-textured hair, wet or dry.

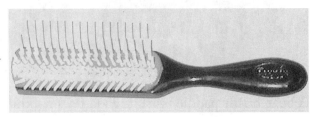

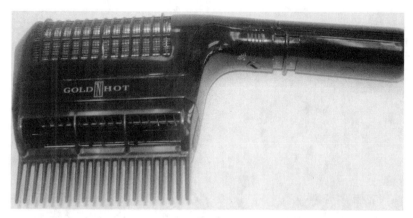

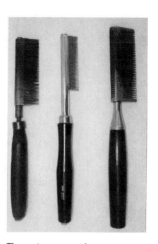

This blow-dryer is not the only type you can use, but it is very easy to work with and helps to straighten the hair while you are drying it.

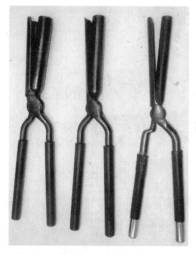

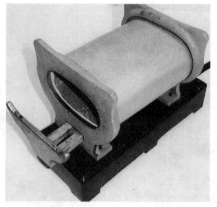

Curling irons come in many sizes and work very well on all types of hair textures. You must learn what degree of heat you should apply when using these irons. The general rule is the softer the hair, the less heat you will need to use.

If you are going to be pressing and curling hair often, you may want to invest in a ceramic stove, which surrounds the pressing comb and the curling iron with heat. These stoves last for years. Of course, if pressing and curling is going to be an occasional thing, you can always use the stovetop to heat up your combs and irons.

Pressing combs can have large, medium, or small teeth, and the teeth can be either curved or straight. The ones shown are designed to go on the stovetop or in a ceramic stove specifically made for pressing combs and curling irons and can get extremely hot, but electric pressing combs are also available. They often have a temperature control and don't get quite as hot.

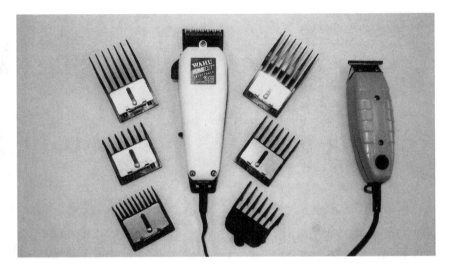

These hair clippers with various-size guards are used to achieve different barber-type cuts.

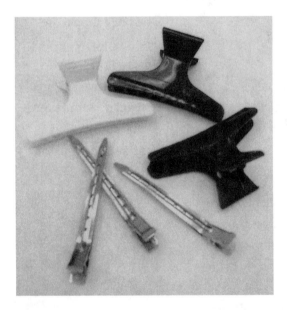

Hair clips are used to hold your child's hair out of the way while you are cutting, relaxing, curling, or blow-drying it.

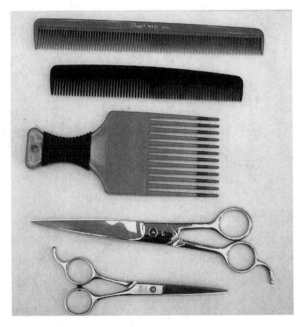

Combs, pick, and scissors are various tools that you will need when cutting your child's hair.

Recommended Reading

Barrick-Hickey, Beth *500 Beauty Solutions: Expert Advice on Hair and Nail Care—What to Buy and How to Use It!* Naperville, Ill: Sourcebooks, 1994.

Elbirt, Paula M.D. *Paula's Good Nutrition Guide for Babies, Toddlers, and Preschoolers.* Cambridge, Mass: Persus Publishing, 2001.

Hofstein, Riquette, with Sallie Baston. *Grow Hair in 12 Weeks: The Natural Healthy Way to Save What You Have and Restore What You Don't in Less Than 1 Hour a Week.* New York: Harmony Books, 1988.

Massey, Lorraine, with Deborah Chiel. *Curly Girl, The Handbook: A Celebration of Curls: How to Cut Them, Care for Them, Love Them, and Set Them Free.* New York: Workman Publishing, 2002.

Sophiscate's BLACK HAIR Styles and Care Guide magazine.

Index